Baby & Me

TOBACCO FREE

*quitting smoking before a child
comes into your life*

D1303307

Laurie Adams & Pamela McColl

Grafton and Scratch Publishers

BABY & ME—TOBACCO FREE

Copyright © Laurie Adams and Pamela McColl 2013

Grafton and Scratch Publishers
www.graftonandscratch.com

Cover photograph credit with thanks to Lina Aidukaite
Book design by Gerilee McBride

Printed and bound in the United States of America

Library and Archives Canada Cataloguing in Publication

Adams, Laurie, 1963–, author
Baby & me tobacco free / Laurie Adams and Pamela McColl.

Issued in print and electronic formats.
ISBN 978-0-9881216-4-5 (pbk.).—ISBN 978-0-9881216-5-2 (pdf).—ISBN 978-0-9881216-6-9 (html)

1. Women—Tobacco use. 2. Pregnant women—Tobacco use. 3. Smoking cessation. I. McColl, Pamela, 1958–, author II. Title. III. Title: Baby and me tobacco free.

HV5746.A32 2013 362.29'6082 C2013-902557-X
C2013-902558-8

"Yesterday is history, tomorrow is mystery, today is a gift."
—*Eleanor Roosevelt*

ABOUT THIS BOOK

The aim of this book is to provide useful information and advice on how to quit smoking for anyone who is either ready to quit or is thinking about doing so before becoming a parent. If you have previously tried to quit but were unsuccessful, this book will not only help you to uncover what has been preventing you from quitting up to this point, but will also help you reach your goal of becoming tobacco-free.

The Baby & Me—Tobacco Free™ Program has proven to be effective in helping thousands of women find lasting success in quitting. This book brings the program to a wider audience than ever before. We hope it will help many parents and their children to live tobacco-free.

"Innovative approaches such as Baby & Me—Tobacco Free™ are for the first time making it possible for us to reduce maternal smoking rates. The potential beneficial impact on society is enormous."—John R. Laird, MD, FACP, FACC, FSCAI Professor of Medicine and Medical Director of the Vascular Center, University of California, Davis Medical Center

ABOUT THE AUTHORS

This book was co-authored to offer readers the combined experiences and expertise of Laurie Adams and Pamela McColl.

LAURIE ADAMS is a certified cessation specialist (board-certified from the University of Pittsburgh) and educator, the creator and Executive Director of the Baby & Me–Tobacco Free Program, and the President/CEO of WELCO Health Education Services. Since 1999, Ms. Adams has contracted with the NY State Tobacco Control Program as the Community Partnerships Program Director for Chautauqua, Cattaraugus, and Allegany (New York). Since 2001, she has provided health and wellness education programs to community agencies and businesses throughout the United States.

PAMELA McCOLL B.A., has placed maternal and child health at the center of her work as a prenatal yoga instructor, labor-support doula, smoking cessation facilitator for close to three decades, and a contented non-smoker. She holds certification in peer counseling from the University of British Columbia, and from the Arizona Healthcare Parternship Maternal and Child Health Tobacco Intervention Skills Training. She is an author, blogger, and award-winning bestselling publisher. Her recent publication of *Twas The Night Before Christmas: Edited by Santa Claus for the benefit of children of the 21st century* (Grafton), the first ever smoke-free edition of the classic tale, created a storm in the national and international media as they took up her call for more to be done to promote tobacco prevention. The book was discussed at length by such noteworthy media outlets as *NBC Nightly News, USA Today, The Guardian, The View, Wall Street Journal, The New York Post* "Bloomberg would love this book", *The Colbert Report,* the *BBC, The Associated Press, The Huffington Post, LA Times,* CBC's *The Current,* and *National Public Radio USA.* (See **www.twasthenightbeforechristmas.ca.**) The edition won three Benjamin Franklin Awards in 2013, a Moonbeam Children's Book Best Book Award in 2012, a Global International E-Book Award also in 2012, and ranked as the #1 bestseller on Amazon.com in the category of 20th century American poetry in December 2012 within 90 days of being released.

Pamela participates on the Western Canadian Action Committee For Smoke Free Movies. She blogs at **www.youcan-stopsmokingnow.com.** You can also follow her on Twitter: **@ twas4kids.** Pamela speaks to parent groups and children regarding tobacco use across North America.

CONTENTS

INTRODUCTION

We start with a question for you: "Would you quit using tobacco and nicotine products if you knew you would achieve lasting success?"

If you answered "Yes, I would," then the material in this book will help you to take the next steps, including planning for success, deciding when to quit, and using tips and strategies to help you follow through on your decision to quit.

If you answered "Not now," we still recommend that you read this book carefully. Some of the questions may spark your curiosity about quitting and you may enjoy reading what other women have to say about the experience of quitting in preparation for motherhood.

If you have tried to quit in the past but found that you were not able to sustain your attempt despite genuinely wanting to, then you stand to gain enormously from the information in this book. We cannot guarantee that you will stop using tobacco products, but we can assure you that you will gain a new perspective on nicotine dependency and the experience of withdrawal and so be in a better position to achieve success.

We strongly believe that there are important reasons for quitting tobacco products at any age and that quitting to better protect children at every stage of their development is highly desirable. But this is your life and you should use this book in a way that suits you. We encourage you to pick and choose from the ideas offered on these pages and to apply those that best suit your current needs. Will you take action to quit the use of tobacco products? That decision rests with you.

In this book we have included answers to questions raised by participants in the Baby & Me—Tobacco Free™ Program. We encourage you to personalize your reading experience by answering the questions we raise and completing the exercises. Have a notebook or file open while you read so you can jot down ideas or suggestions that resonate with you. A section at the back of the book deals specifically with quit plans and will be useful to you when you craft your own action strategy. If you have already quit smoking and want an answer to a specific question, you can use the index to find the appropriate subject and corresponding pages.

AN IMPORTANT DECISION

The material in this book is intended for parents-to–be but will also be relevant to any family member or caregiver who wants to quit tobacco for the sake of the new family. The prospect of parenthood brings a new importance to making healthy lifestyle choices to best meet the challenges that come with caring for newborns and young children. Opportunity knocks for positive change when you are starting a family, whether you are pregnant, becoming a parent through adoption or fostering, or joining an existing family that includes children.

It is a well-established fact that continuing to smoking during pregnancy poses serious immediate and lasting health risks to both the baby and the mother. Ongoing exposure to second- and third-hand smoke increases the risk of harm.

Pregnancy is an excellent time to quit.

- Your quit effort will be supported because many—in fact, probably most—people understand the consequences of continuing to use tobacco products and the risks of second-hand smoke.
- The total restriction of alcohol and the reduction or elimination of caffeine, common smoking triggers, will help you quit.
- When pregnant, you will be focused on having a healthy pregnancy and will be paying attention to eating well and getting adequate rest and regular exercise. These healthy lifestyle choices will assist your quit effort.
- You will benefit from increased access to cessation information and resources. Many people will be ready and willing to offer you pregnancy tips and suggestions. A midwife, doctor, nurse, healthcare worker, doula, prenatal instructor, family members, and friends are all people with whom you can discuss pregnancy-specific concerns, including the subject of quitting tobacco. Other pregnant women can be very helpful and you may find someone who is interested in becoming a "quitting buddy."
- People who smoke may refrain from lighting up around you, making it easier for you to quit and remain smoke-free.

Choosing to quit as you prepare to welcome a child into your life is one of the most important decisions you will ever make in terms of taking care of your health and the health of your child.

The positive effects of this one lifestyle change will ripple out to touch every aspect of your life.

If you make quitting tobacco a priority, there will be immediate and lasting benefits to you and your baby.

- Your sense of taste and smell will return, and food will become more enjoyable and satisfying. You may find yourself rejecting junk food as tasteless.
- With more money at your disposal, now that you aren't spending on tobacco products, you will be able to buy better quality food.
- You will have more money to buy the things you will need for the baby.
- Your body will have more oxygen. You may enjoy exercise more.
- After you quit smoking you will probably have significantly lower levels of anxiety than you had when you were smoking.
- You can now take a real break at work or at home, not just a break to smoke.
- By achieving this one important goal, your confidence will increase.

Here are a couple of questions to get things started.

QUESTION 1: Which one of these statements best describes your current use of tobacco/nicotine products?

1. I have thought about quitting but I am not ready yet.
2. I want to quit soon.
3. I have not decided.
4. I don't want to quit.

5. I quit smoking recently but I feel urges.
6. I quit smoking and I am sure I won't start again.
7. I quit smoking but I am not sure I will make this permanent.

Or describe in your own words your current use of tobacco products (use a journal or open a file to complete this answer).

Write in today's date here: _____

Idea: When you have finished reading this book, come back here and ask yourself these questions again. Note if anything has changed.

QUESTION 2: Do you know what is preventing you from quitting tobacco? If you do not know, leave this question for now and come back to it if the reason comes to you as you read this book.

BABY & ME—TOBACCO FREE: MAKING A DIFFERENCE

In spite of everything you know about why you need to stop using tobacco, you are probably in the same position as 95% of people who smoke.

The vast majority of smokers wish they could quit but do not know how to do it successfully.

An estimated 30% of women who regularly use tobacco before they become pregnant will quit during a pregnancy. This is higher than the quit rate given for the general population. But these statistics also tell us that approximately 70% of North American women who smoke will continue to do so during a pregnancy.

Of the women who do quit during pregnancy, many do not remain tobacco-free. An estimated 25% of women who quit during pregnancy return to using tobacco products before giving birth, 50% return to using tobacco products by four months postpartum, 60% return to using tobacco products by six months postpartum, and between 70% and 90% go back to using tobacco products within the first year of giving birth.

The Baby & Me—Tobacco Free™ Program, which began in 2002 in New York State, undertook an extensive research project from 2006 to 2009. The research was funded by the New York State Control Program and was conducted under the direction of WELCO Health Education Services and the evaluation team at Bassett Research Institute, Cooperstown, New York. The results were published in *Maternal and Child Health Journal* in January 2011.

> Our formal evaluation of this program demonstrated that it was effective in helping pregnant women quit smoking and stay quit. This cessation program saves lives, and greatly benefits the health of a new mom, her baby and her other children as well as reduces costs associated with preterm birth and NICU hospitalization. —Dr. Anne Gadomski, MD, Senior Research Scientist/Attending Pediatrician, Bassett Medical Center, Cooperstown, NY, and Associate Professor, Department of Pediatrics, Columbia University, New York, NY.

ABOUT BABY & ME—TOBACCO FREE

The Baby & Me—Tobacco Free™ Program brings women together with specialized counselors who offer positive reinforcement and factual information, and answer questions about quitting in a non-judgmental and respectful way. Today the program enrolls thousands of pregnant women through collaborations with local family programs, obstetric and prenatal clinics, and The Prenatal Care Assistance Program, and by physician referral.

Participants attend four monthly prenatal counseling sessions, and stay with the program for between six months and one year postpartum. The participants are asked at the outset about their current tobacco product use and their level of interest in quitting. As a condition of enrollment in the program, the participant is asked to commit to making a serious quit effort, to set a quit date, and to attend the sessions and follow the program's guidelines. A unique aspect of the program is the eligibility of postpartum participants to receive vouchers for free diapers if they test tobacco-free at each postpartum appointment. The program is currently offered nationwide throughout the United States. In 2005, the program received a Model Practice Award by the National Association of City and County Health Officials.

Laurie Adams, Executive Director of the Baby & Me—Tobacco Free™ Program, provides a certified cessation training seminar for agencies that want to implement the program. The facilitators learn the core components of administering the program. The Baby & Me—Tobacco Free™ Program protocols are evidenced-based and geared toward the needs of the pregnant woman. The trained facilitators learn how to talk to their clients about the stages of change, how to set a quit date, how to ask for a tobacco-free home and car, and how to be prepared for life without cigarettes or other tobacco products. The training provides key support from the Clinical Practice Guidelines for Treating Tobacco Dependence (2008 update).

WHAT BABY & ME—TOBACCO FREE PARTICIPANTS SAY ABOUT THE PROGRAM

"*I could never have stayed quit without the program and the support. I learned how to quit and how to ask for a smoke-free home and car to protect the baby and me. The free diapers were wonderful, but I really had much more of a reward by having a healthy baby and protecting her when she came home from the hospital.*" —Krystal M.

"*The toughest time for me was when I got really stressed out. But I learned that stress happens to everyone and non-smokers don't smoke when they're stressed. I had to work through it and find other ways to manage my stress. The program really helped.*" —Alicia W.

"*Even though some of my family wasn't always supportive, I insisted on a smoke-free home. I learned that there's no safe level of second-hand smoke.*" —Laura K.

"*Thank you for the program. I needed the positive reinforcement to quit and stay quit. My boyfriend smokes and now it smells so bad. I don't want to smell like that ever again.*" —Jennifer L.

"*I was worried about going back to smoking after the baby was born but I learned that cigarettes' chemicals go into breast milk and I wanted to nurse. The program really helped.*" —Jordan G.

"Apathy can be overcome by enthusiasm, and enthusiasm can only be aroused by two things: First, an ideal, which takes the imagination by storm, and second, a definite intelligible plan for carrying that ideal into practice." —Arnold J. Toynbee

PART ONE:
THIS BOOK CAN MAKE A DIFFERENCE

"The success of self-help books in our time reflects a constructive desire on the part of people to take responsibility for their own mental health and spiritual development. However, most such books also focus on teaching us what is wrong with ourselves and then telling us how we can get better. Just as with a computer, we may not need to be fixed; we simply may need to learn to understand what we have going for us and how to use it in the current stage of our journey."
—Carol S. Pearson, *The Hero Within.*

The most significant message of this book is that you can and must use your own inherent strengths to find your way to a tobacco-free life. Escaping your dependency on tobacco products has everything to do with using the powers you already possess to instigate change. It has everything to do with first of all believing that it is possible to quit, rebuilding trust in your own abilities, and affording yourself compassion. Finding your way clear of tobacco products also involves placing the burden of blame where it belongs—that is, not with you but with the individuals who run the tobacco industry. Armed with new information and a re-evaluation of tobacco products, it is absolutely possible to set yourself free.

"To love a person is to see all of their magic, and to remind them of it when they have forgotten." —Anonymous

Many years ago I was training to be a labor-support doula. One day in class the instructor made a comment: "If a client mentions that she would like to hear the mellow songstress Enya while she is in labor, it would be best to offer her further information on the birthing process."

The instructor emphasized that although the doula should offer techniques to help a woman in labor remain calm and focused, it was also important to be realistic about the more challenging stages of labor. She continued to explain that labor is work. It is, of course, a labor of love, but it also demands a great deal of energy. Having a realistic outlook on birthing gives a woman time to consider various options that could help her remain strong and confident as labor progresses.

Over the past several decades prenatal education has gone through many changes. It is wonderful that we are seeing programs incorporating meditation and yoga, with an emphasis on body awareness, the mind-body relationship, and the importance of preparing and understanding the birth process.

When a woman comes to me as a new client in my doula practice and she tells me that she wants to have a natural childbirth or that she wants to quit smoking before she starts a family, we will discuss the steps she can take to increase the likelihood of that hope becoming a reality.

➤ WHETHER QUITTING SMOKING OR HAVING A BABY NATURALLY, IT LIKELY WILL TAKE MORE THAN WISHFUL THINKING TO GET THE LASTING RESULTS YOU DESIRE.

I first met Laurie Adams in New Orleans at a tobacco prevention conference in early 2012. At that time I had started writing a book based on my direct experience with successfully overcoming addictions and on my work as a labor-support doula, specializing in maternal smoking cessation. I was very impressed with the results Laurie was achieving with women from all over the United States. Often, all these women needed was solid, practical advice combined with information about the tobacco products they were using and a healthy dose of inspiration. Laurie and I decided to collaborate to bring our combined perspectives and experiences together to better serve women ready to make this lifestyle change in preparation for parenthood.

HOW I QUIT

Having managed to quit a variety of "off-limits" substances during all my pregnancies, I knew the sweet feeling of success that comes with actually doing what you have committed to do instead of just talking or thinking about it. Unfortunately, my success would inevitably be fleeting, and I invariably found myself settling back into my pre-pregnancy ways. I was essentially at war with myself. I found myself constantly worrying about the potential consequences of my choices. I would dwell not only on the money I was spending but also on the time and energy I was wasting in a fight I was worried I might never win.

My world changed.

To this day I cannot imagine ever lighting up a cigarette, and it takes no effort on my part to be a non-smoker. How did I manage that? I found lasting success when I found the answer to a question that was put to me by a friend who also wanted to quit but did not know how to go about it.

My friend confided that she wished she could remain pregnant all the time because it was only when she was expecting that she could keep herself from smoking. My imagination got the better of me and I started to dream about what it might be like to live out such a wish, living in a state of eternal maternity, being a real-life Mother Goose. Mother Goose, as far as I recall, ended up with so many children that she did not have a clue what to do and lived in a shoe of all places. I concluded that this was indeed rather a drastic way to stay off nicotine. My friend's comment was made in jest but her frustration was coming through loud and clear and it had an all too familiar ring to it. She told me that she held off from smoking during two pregnancies but for some reason she could not find the same success in a non-pregnant state. She and I agreed that the whole process was utterly exhausting and also very strange.

HOW DO WE EXPLAIN THE OCCURRENCE OF SUCCESSFUL QUITTING?

How do you explain the fact that some—but not all—people are able to spontaneously quit using addictive substances and to stay free of them while others struggle? And why are these same people only able to quit at specific times in their life?

For example, a woman enters a medical clinic and is told she is pregnant. These few words make her able to quit addictive substances in that moment. How do we explain this? What does it say about addiction?

Some people are quick to say that in this type of case, the

sudden ability to spontaneously quit must be due to concern for the baby. However, this does not explain why some women, in the same situation with the same level of concern for their babies, do not find immediate success. We need to dig a little deeper to fully understand the curious case of the spontaneous quitter.

"Inside the soul our god-given gifts, natural talents, and endless imagination waits to awaken and be put to greater use." —Michael Meade

A DISCOVERY
Spontaneous quitting is ignited by the instantaneous and remarkable power of the imagination making room for something new to take hold, offering you something new to believe while sweeping away a string of old beliefs that no longer fit. The mysterious case of the spontaneous quitter does not tell us that addictions are not real but rather that the experience of quitting can be radically altered in a moment of time. This is very encouraging news.

THE PROCESS
After you have read through this book, completed the exercises, and spent time reflecting on your own beliefs about the use of tobacco products, one of two things will likely happen. You will either find your way off tobacco products relatively smoothly or you will wake up on your designated quit date and still be uneasy about what lies ahead. In the case of this second outcome, the tips, strategies, and quit plans you have made will be useful

tools to meet challenges as you set out on your journey. However, both outcomes will get you where you are headed—safely away from tobacco. The more you can break down the beliefs that are holding you to tobacco and nicotine, the smoother the process will be for you.

Having a plan in place before you launch a quit attempt is key to success in the case of the second scenario but the same preparatory steps will influence your quitting success in either scenario.

"The most beautiful things we can experience are the mysterious. It is the source of all true art and science." —Albert Einstein

I STARTED WHEN I WAS A KID

How old were you when you started using tobacco products?

How old were you when you became a regular tobacco-product consumer?

Do you know why you started?

Many people start smoking before the age of 18. However, data released early in 2013 revealed an increase in the number of people who started smoking after the age of 20, with 15% of women taking up smoking after age 25. The data were based on a survey of Americans between 1997 and 2004, and the findings are in stark contrast to previous data that showed virtually all smokers starting in their teen years.

The data, reported in the *New England Journal of Medicine* in January 2013, also provided new findings on the specific risks for women of long-term use of tobacco products and the benefits of cessation at any age.

➤ **CULTURAL INFLUENCES**

2013: MUSIC VIDEO FOR *SUIT AND TIE* SHOWS SINGER JUSTIN TIMBERLAKE SMOKING.

FEBRUARY 2013: SINGER RIHANNA IS SHOWN SMOKING A CIGARETTE IN A PHOTO-SHOOT FOR *ROLLING STONE MAGAZINE.*

MAY 2013: MAGAZINE COVERS FEATURE SMOKING: *ROLLING STONE* HAS SINGER BRUNO MARS AND *ESQUIRE* MAGAZINE HAS ACTOR LEONARDO DICAPRIO—BOTH ARE DEPICTED WITH CIGARETTES

MARCH 9, 2011: KATE MOSS SMOKES ON THE RUNWAY DURING THE LOUIS VUITTON FASHION SHOW IN PARIS.

LYRICS OF THE FAITHLESS SONG *MISS U LESS* INCLUDE THE WORDS "I LOVE THE WAY YOU SMOKE."

IN THE MOVIE *GANGSTER SQUAD,* STARRING EMMA STONE AND RYAN GOSLING, EMMA STONE IS SHOWN SMOKING.

IN THE MOVIE *SKYFALL,* BÉRÉNICE MARLOHE'S CHARACTER IS SHOWN SMOKING.

MAKING CHANGE HAPPEN

At some point, you accepted the idea that tobacco was worth experimenting with. You may have imagined that by using these products you would appear sexier or be more popular. Whatever your reasons for starting, tied into them was the notion that smoking would do something for you—there would be benefits.

Your vivid imagination was influenced by the advertising machine of the tobacco industry and a social culture that reinforced the use of tobacco products. In viewing the covers of current magazines or recently released music videos, it is apparent that the projected glamorous image of smoking has never really died and that young adults continue to be persuaded to use tobacco products by powers behind the scenes.

THE POWER OF IMAGINATION

Now that you want to make a change, you can once again use the significant powers of your imagination to get yourself off these substances. You are not being asked to get out of your situation by imagining the worst of possible outcomes. In fact, you are going to be asked to do the complete opposite.

Exercise #1: What does success look like to you?

Close your eyes and dream of an answer to each of the following questions. You can return to this page as you read through this book. There is no need to rush. Take your time. Bring success into focus and define it in your own terms. You can also write your answers in your journal or file.

What does success in quitting look or feel like to you?

Examples:

Success would mean I could stop hiding.

Success would mean I wouldn't have to worry all the time.

Success would mean more money for other things I need.

Success would be great.

Success would mean I have done an important thing to protect my health and the health of my family.

What could you do today that would have an impact on success in the future?

Examples:

Success would mean that I set a day to quit.

Success would mean that I talked to my partner about making a decision to quit and he decided to quit with me.

What does success look like one week from now?
Example:
Success would mean my car is smoke-free in one week from now and in two weeks will be clear of third-hand smoke residue and safe for my baby.

What does success look like one month from now?
Example:
Success would mean telling everyone at work that I quit and they congratulate me.
Success would mean that I saved enough from not smoking this month to buy some of the things on the list of items I need for the new baby.

What does success look like one year from now?
Example:
Success would be that I saved enough money from not smoking to book a family holiday in the sun.

What does success look like five years from now?
Example:
Success would be looking back with pride and realizing that I did this for my family and myself.

What does success look like ten years from now?
Examples:
Success would be when I have had three pregnancies and have managed to remain tobacco-free.
Success would be when my teenager came to me and I could

help them not get started on drugs because I knew about the experience of addiction and withdrawal first-hand.

Once you have a clearer picture of what success looks or feels like for you, write down any ideas or answers that come to mind. It could be a word or a simple phrase or a sentence.

Are there any things that you think need to happen for you to achieve success?

Does someone else need to do something?
Example:
Success would require my husband to also quit.

Does something specific need to be put in place before you can achieve success?
Write down anything at all that comes to mind. Be aware that this is where excuses may start to emerge. Remember that there are no wrong answers. The goal is to find out what is holding you back. If you don't have anything to write that is also perfectly okay.
Examples:
I need to find a way to handle the stress in my life.
I need to know that I won't gain weight if I quit.

Exercise #2: How would quitting affect your life?
Draw a circle and divide it into 12 sections. Label each section with a part of your life: family, friends, work, spirituality, exercise, finances, health, pets, travel, home, hobbies, or any other areas where you focus your attention. Spend a few minutes considering each of these parts of your life and how successfully

quitting tobacco use would affect each of these areas. Allow your imagination free rein.

"Imagination is more powerful than knowledge." —Albert Einstein

We use our powers of imagination to review information. We take what we think will work and construct our worlds accordingly. We are going to look at some of the beliefs you held when you were a youth about the use of tobacco products. We suggest you hold on only to those beliefs that still have value in your current life.

Do you remember any of your beliefs about tobacco products that got you started on tobacco use? Do any of these beliefs hold true today?

Do your friends still think it is acceptable to smoke? Do your friends or family think it is okay to smoke while pregnant?

Do they see you as a daring risk-taker, a rebel, or sexier or more attractive because you smoke? Circumstances change and, with a little work, our beliefs can be adapted to fit new situations through the power of imagination and knowledge.

MESSAGES ABOUT TOBACCO PRODUCTS

From a very young age you have been exposed to the tobacco industry. In the United States alone, tobacco companies spend more than $1 million an hour on marketing their products. The result? More than 80% of underage smokers smoke cigarettes that are among the top three most heavily advertised brands.

The badness of smoking was constituted by more than its effect on health. Embedded in the cigarette were the complex historical meanings of rebellion idleness, independence and attraction. All kids were told smoking was bad—and was only for adults—who created, in part, its impressive appeal. And this appeal was anything but natural. It was the studied and meticulous invention of the industry that would come to understand—and exploit—critical aspects of motivation, psychology, and human biology. This book marks my attempt to resolve a child's paradox—a paradox of pandemic proportions. (Allan M. Brandt in his introduction to *The Cigarette Century: The Rise, Fall and Deadly Persistence of the Product that Defined America.*)

An estimated 2/3 of children experiment with tobacco products. Unfortunately, you were one of the people who bought into the idea that smoking was the thing to do. Just like the movie stars and music idols who continue to present the use of tobacco as glamorous, you bought into the myth of tobacco.

A child's exposure to smoking on screen makes the most difference in how likely they are to start smoking.

From 2010 to 2011, tobacco incidents per youth-rated film jumped 34%, according to a report by the US Centers for Disease Control and Prevention.

On May 8, 2012, the National Association of Attorneys General (NAAG) sent a letter, signed by 38 state and territorial attorneys general, to 10 movie studios, alerting them to the need to eliminate tobacco depictions in youth-rated film productions. They wrote in part:

- This is a colossal, preventable tragedy. There are specific meaningful steps your studio can and should take to reduce this harm substantially. A point we made to studio nearly five years ago bears repeating: each time the industry releases another movie that depicts smoking, it does so with the full knowledge of the harm it will bring to children who watch it.

The U.S. Surgeon General's Report of March 8, 2012, *Preventing Tobacco Use Among Youth and Young Adults*, stated that "the evidence is sufficient to conclude that there is a casual relationship between depictions of smoking in the movies and the initiation of smoking among young people."

*"Teens that see the most smoking in movies are three times more likely to start smoking than those who see the least." —*Dartmouth Medical School

It would have been so much simpler to have never started but that was yesterday and yesterday has gone. Today you are facing a decision: you can accept your life and keep things as they are, or you can decide to make a serious attempt at quitting.

Arrival—A Poem

If you have arrived at a place
Where you see quitting a substance
As an insurmountable problem
You may choose to run away
There is no reason
No matter how profound that will call you back
You have arrived at the conclusion you will defy the odds
Deny the statistics
You are still running but in the opposite direction
You can choose to challenge both directions
You can choose to consider
There might be just one more
Possible direction left to explore

P.M.

PART TWO: HOW DO I QUIT SMOKING BEFORE A CHILD ARRIVES IN MY LIFE?

Q#9   "Is cutting down a good strategy for quitting?" (p. 56)

Q#10 "Smoking helps me handle stress. What will happen when I quit?" (p. 58)

Q#11 "I know about the risks but I can't get through a day without lighting up. How do other pregnant women find it so easy?" (p. 64)

Q#12 "Is it true that nicotine is the hardest drug to get off?" (p. 65)

Q#13 "Does smoking help with weight loss?" (p. 67)

Q#14 "Smoking helps me go to sleep at night. Now I am pregnant but I haven't decided if I am going to quit or not. I like it." (p.75)

Q#15 "I know women who use marijuana when they are pregnant and my friend told me it would help with morning sickness. What do you think?" (p. 77)

Q#16 "I feel like a cigarette. Now what do I do?" (p. 77)

Q#17 "How do I handle going out with my friends and not lighting up again? What will happen when I start drinking again?" (p. 79)

Q#18 "I couldn't quit for the reason of protecting my own health. Is low self-esteem why I can't quit?" (p. 80)

Q#19 "What can I do to improve my chances of success? I don't want to waste any time now that I know I am pregnant." (p. 81)

Q#20 "When I quit, for how long will the cravings continue?" (p. 84)

Q#21 "Do strategies and distractions work?" (p. 86)

Q#22 "Why is it that I sometimes I feel like I have plenty of willpower and at other times I don't feel like I have enough to keep me from smoking?" (p. 88)

Q#23 "Some of the things I have read scare me. Where can I get good information that won't make me feel terrible?" (p. 90)

Q#24 "I heard that I should quit gradually or it could be too much of a shock for the baby. Is that true?" (p. 92)

Q#25 "My mother smoked during all of her pregnancies and we all turned out okay. Why do I need to quit?" (p. 92)

Q#26 "Will trying to quit now that I am pregnant put too much pressure on me and possibly cause depression? I have been depressed in the past." (p. 99)

Q#27 "When is it okay to return to alcohol after giving birth? I also want to limit the binge drinking I was doing before I became pregnant." (p. 102)

Q#28 "I have switched to e-cigarettes. Is that a good idea?" (p. 104)

Q#29 "I am facing problems in my life right now so I can't deal with quitting." (p. 106)

Q#30 "How can finding someone to help support me make a difference?" (p. 108)

Q#31 "How can I respond to criticism that I have not been able to quit?" (p. 111)

Q#32 "What are the best reasons for quitting?" (p. 113)

Q#33 "How can I get other people who will be around the baby to understand the risks of second-hand and third-hand smoke?" (p. 114)

Q#34 "I have no self-control and don't believe I can do this long-term." (p. 117)

Q#35 "What can I do or say that will help my dad? He wants to quit but the topic makes him uncomfortable." (p. 120)

Q#36 "My mom has never smoked and has no patience for anyone who does. What can I say that will help her to understand what I am going through?" (p. 121)

Q#1 "I WANTED TO QUIT BEFORE GETTING PREGNANT BUT COULDN'T. I AM STILL SMOKING AND SO ASHAMED THAT SOMETIMES I CRY WHEN I SMOKE."

If you used tobacco products prior to finding out that you were pregnant or you are still using them in a current pregnancy, please treat yourself with compassion. Let's agree to not make things more challenging by descending in a self-loathing downward slide. It can be a treacherous and slippery slope. Note that this is not a suggestion that you attempt to deny any feelings that are presenting themselves. It is a recommendation that you catch yourself in as wide a net as possible and simply hang out there, while you give yourself a break from your battle and read through these pages.

Idea: Making changes in your life.

If you want to make a big change in your life, it might be good to start with a small change first. Get started by making a positive change to your daily routine:

- Change your hairstyle.
- Change your perfume.
- Buy a new purse.
- Go to a new place to shop.
- Walk a new route.
- Make a new friend.
- See Shaping Up for a Healthy Pregnancy on page 141.
- Start writing in a journal.

Slow down and prepare to listen to your thoughts and feelings.

Escaping the burden of self-blame.

In the 21st century people who continue to smoke are subject to severe marginalization while the people behind the tobacco industry peddle their product on the global market. The World Health Organization estimates that, in this century alone, 1 billion people will die a premature, tobacco-product–related death and countless more will have their quality of life affected or destroyed by diseases related to the use of tobacco products. Healthcare systems around the world will be tested in the coming decades by the tobacco industry's advances like never before and there are individuals who need to be held accountable.

Information coming out of the Centers for Disease Control and Prevention (CDC) shows that worldwide, tobacco products cause more than 5 million deaths per year, and current trends suggest that tobacco use will cause more than 8 million deaths annually by 2030. CDC data identifies smoking as responsible for about one in five deaths annually in the United States. Tobacco products cost the U.S. healthcare system $96 billion annually with an additional $10 billion in expenditures related to the damage caused by exposure to second-hand smoke.

The tobacco epidemic.

The August 2012 results of the largest-ever study on global tobacco use, The Global Adult Tobacco Study, showed that an estimated 49% of men and 11% of women in developing countries smoke and/or use smokeless tobacco. It was also noted that females are starting to smoke at increasingly young ages.

The tobacco industry.
• While populations were being addicted, the cigarette

manufacturers were also engaged in an ongoing campaign to convince legislators and the public that, as legal enterprises marketing legal, normal products, they are entitled to be treated in the same manner as other companies. In brief, the industry has hidden its predatory marketing behind a veil of normalcy and rationalized its epidemic on "free choice" rhetoric and fraud. (TID) Tobacco Industry Denormalization is a health strategy that places the responsibility for the tobacco epidemic where it belongs, on the corporate misbehaviour rather than on the individual misjudgement. TID puts a spotlight on corporate fraud negligence and their failure to warn, rather than on teenage miscalculations of the risks of addiction or on the failure of youth to recognize that they are the targets of predatory marketing by adults.

- The tobacco industry's message is unmistakable. There is no need to worry because the more than 20 terminal tobacco diseases that constitute the tobacco epidemic are brought to you by a "legal," normal industry selling a "legal," normal product. Tobacco industry products will kill one out of two of their long-term users. That's a death rate of 50 percent! Other drugs would be pulled off the market if the risk of death from use was even a small fraction of the risk of using tobacco. (Garfield Mahood, Executive Director, 1976–2011, Non-Smokers' Rights Association, Canada.)

In *The Economist*, October 2, 2000, Dr. Gro Harlem Brundtland, in his capacity as Director-General of the World Health Organization, compared the role of the tobacco industry in creating health problems to that of the mosquito in causing malaria. "Both are blood-sucking, disease-spreading parasites."

U.S. Judge H. Lee Sarokin remarked on the "industry wide conspiracy to accomplish all of the foregoing [efforts to deceive the public] in callous, wanton, willful and reckless disregard for the health of consumers in an effort to maintain sales and profits ... [a conspiracy] vast in its scope, devious in its purpose and devastating in its results."

Once you understand how you have been used by the tobacco industry you can devote your energies, possibly fueled by outrage, to deciding whether or not to put everything into making a serious effort to quit.

If you decide to quit, it is recommended that you put the date in writing in your quit plan. When your quit day arrives, you will take the first step to becoming tobacco-free in time to welcome a new child into your life.

Q#2 "I TRIED TO QUIT BEFORE AND IT DIDN'T WORK. NOW WHAT DO I DO?"

Finding your way off tobacco products is more complicated than simply ridding your physical body of the drug nicotine. Otherwise, more people would successfully quit on their very first attempt. Did you know that the vast majority of people who succeed at quitting used the "cold turkey" approach? Did you know that it took them multiple attempts before they actually quit?

Facts about withdrawal.

People experience withdrawal, the physical effects of ridding the body of nicotine, very differently. Some people report having few noticeable symptoms, however hard that may be to believe. The process of withdrawal is also significantly affected by the psychological aspect of quitting—and again, the experience varies greatly. The more you fear quitting, the greater will be the chance that you will experience distressing physical and psychological symptoms.

- It takes an estimated 48 to 96 hours to be physically clear of nicotine.
- Withdrawal symptoms usually start between 30 minutes and two hours after the last cigarette was been put out.
- Symptoms most frequently peak two to three days after going tobacco-free.
- On average, a single physical withdrawal craving lasts one to three minutes and occurs, on average, six times a day for a couple of days.

A question for you: On a scale of 1 to 10, with 1 meaning "I don't want to quit in the next two weeks" and 10 being "I have decided I am ready," how would you rate your attitude to making a serious quit attempt in the next few weeks?

Put your selected number between 1 and 10 here: _____

If you are unsure, you don't need to have a yes or no answer right now. Start slowly, taking baby steps with the help of the LOL (Less or Later) strategy. Smoke less often and, when you do, smoke less of a cigarette. Try this strategy for a few days and then rate your attitude again. Have you given a different answer? Confidence thrives on repeated success.

To effectively use the LOL strategy, write down how many cigarettes you are currently smoking each day and then set a specific lesser amount for the next seven days. Write down your progress. Use the "smoke later" strategy by setting a specific time to push off the decision to light up again. For example, instead of smoking during your afternoon break, tell yourself you will make it until after work to decide whether or not you want a cigarette. When you have reached your targeted reduction of cigarettes for the determined number of days, reward yourself. Plan the rewards ahead of time: book a massage or movie date with a friend. During the week, keep your eyes on the prize.

Tip: The Five "D's" strategy for handling withdrawal.
You may find it helpful to write these five ideas out and keep them close at hand.

1. Delay.
2. Drink water or other beverage you like.
3. Do something else.
4. Deep-breathe.
5. Discuss. Have people with whom you can discuss quitting available by phone, social media, or email.

Although millions of people have successfully quit smoking and their success has been the subject of extensive study, it remains impossible for anyone to provide the specific steps that will lead to success in quitting smoking. You will quit in your own time and in your own way.

"Checking yourself out, noticing how you feel, and observing your thoughts without buying into them, is a profoundly significant moment. It will give you the power to act from a resourceful, skillful place."
—Sally Kempton

Q#3 "HOW DO I CHOOSE A QUIT DATE?"

If you are ready to commit to a quit attempt, set a day to quit within the next two weeks. This will give you time to prepare your quit plan and to finish reading this book. Write down any thoughts or feelings that you have about setting a date in your quit plan.

Why not just quit tomorrow?

Let's forget about quitting smoking for a minute and consider a different scenario. If you were to set a goal to perform a high dive, something you had never done before, what do you think your dive would look like if you were to attempt it later today with no preparation?

If you set a date to do it in two weeks, you have time to get a few tips, learn a few things, maybe see how other people have done it, or get advice. With some practice and some ideas you won't end up either freaking out at the end of the board or scrambling down without making an attempt—or even worse, plunging off the board and then remembering you can't swim.

Preparing a quit date two weeks away works in the same way. Two weeks is a good amount of time to make the necessary plans and get yourself prepared—maybe not perfectly prepared, but at least better prepared than you are right now.

Try not to find reasons to delay your decision. If you wait for a stress-free period to quit, you could find yourself waiting for a long time. Picking a day in two weeks' time is a simple and effective decision-making strategy.

A little gem of yoga wisdom:

If you attend a yoga class and there is a note on the door

that reads "Quiet Please: Yoga Class in Progress," do everyone a favor and flip it over.

You cannot tell the world to stop and be quiet while you get your meditation or whatever else you are trying to do in your life right. You can only control what happens on your "mat" and, if in the sublime moment of relaxation, someone or something interrupts your space thank them for helping you to deepen your practice.

There is no such thing as the perfect time to quit. You can and should prepare the way but expect interruptions. Life has a way of showing up. Make the proper, but not necessarily perfect, preparations and then meet your quit date.

Q#4 "WHAT IS A QUIT PLAN?"

A quit plan is simply a written plan of action outlining how you plan to quit smoking. It is important to include as much personal detail as possible in your quit plan.

By preparing a quit plan ahead of making a serious effort to quit, you significantly improve your chances of success. It helps you plan and strategize for different outcomes. Adding details to your plan will make it a valuable part of the quitting process. Suggestions for creating a quit plan are provided at the back of this book, along with a review of key questions and exercises. You will need to purchase a notebook or open a file on your computer where you can make the necessary notes and record your preparation.

A quit plan should include the following:

1. A definition of what success would look and feel like.

2. A written statement about your commitment to quitting and the date you will quit.
3. The benefits of quitting.
4. Your personal reasons for quitting.
5. Your support list, identifying people who can help you in your quit effort.
6. Strategies for handling stressors and triggers.
7. How you will manage withdrawal symptoms.
8. What it means to you to live a tobacco-free life.

Q#5 "WILL I QUIT?"
Exercise #3: "Will I quit?"
Take a moment to write answers to the questions below. There are no wrong answers and no one else will ever see what you have written unless you want them to. Just write what seems true for you. Write the answers here or in your journal.

"Will I quit?"

How would your heart answer this question?

How would your head answer this question?

How would your gut answer?

Review your answers.

Do you have any concerns around the idea of quitting?

List any words that come up in response to the idea of quitting.

Q#6 "WHAT METHODS HAVE SUCCESSFUL QUITTERS USED?"
Over 90% of successful quitters achieved success with an unaided spontaneous quit attempt, or what is commonly referred to as

"going cold turkey." The people who found success with cold turkey did not just forget to smoke one day. It had nothing to do with the full moon, New Year's Eve, or wanting a fresh start one Monday morning. Something fundamentally changed for these individuals, and it was only then that they could free themselves.

Here is what people have had to say about spontaneous quitting.

"It was time."

"It is day three...and I'm hanging in there."

"It is one year and I am celebrating."

Before you give serious thought to going for a white-knuckle attempt at cold turkey, you should know about this method's chances of success.

A single attempt at quitting the use of tobacco products by going cold turkey has been proven to have a success rate of just 3.4%.

So how did 90% of quitters achieve success if the average success rate is 3.4% for a single attempt?

On average it will take an individual between 5.3 and 11.1 serious single attempts before they quit for good. The people who succeed get there by trying over and over again. Unfortunately, most people give up after numerous failed attempts and never go back to trying. It is very important to build an action plan before making a quit attempt to prevent repeated and exhausting defeat after defeat.

"At some level, "this might not work" is at the heart of all important projects, of everything new and worth doing. And it can paralyze us into inaction, into watering down our art and into failing to ship. This might not work is either a curse, something that you labour under or it's a blessing, a chance to fly, and do work you never thought possible." —Seth Godin

Q#7 "ARE NICOTINE REPLACEMENT THERAPIES EFFECTIVE? CAN I USE THEM WHILE PREGNANT OR WILL THEY HARM THE BABY?"

Since the mid-1980s, nicotine replacement therapy (NRT) has been marketed as a smoking cessation aid. The one-year success rates for NRT products, taken from the Cochrane Reviews, are 6.2% for the nicotine patch and 5.7% for the nicotine gum. What is particularly interesting is that, unlike cold turkey which can produce positive results after repeated attempts, a second attempt at using NRT reduces the chances of success. In some studies, success from a second attempt has been shown to be zero.

The manufacturers of NRT products do not make any claims about long-term abstinence and openly state that the products are designed to assist with withdrawal symptoms. There seems to be a general misconception that NRT will help smokers to quit when that is not what they were designed to do. They may play a role in harm reduction.

Early in 2012 the Harvard School of Public Health issued the following statement:

> Nicotine replacement therapies (NRTs) designed to help people stop smoking, specifically nicotine patches and nicotine gum, do not appear to be effective in helping smokers quit long-term, even when combined with smoking cessation counseling, according to a new study by researchers at Harvard School of Public Health (HSPH) and the University of Massachusetts Boston. The researchers found no difference in relapse rates among those who used NRT for more than six weeks, with or without professional counseling. No difference in quitting success with use of NRT was found for either heavy or light smokers.

The study demonstrates that using NRT is no more effective in helping people stop smoking cigarettes in the long-term than quitting unaided.

NRT is not recommended in the presence of special circumstances, including the use by populations for which there is insufficient evidence of effectiveness: people who smoke less than 10 cigarettes per day, adolescents (under 18 years of age), pregnant women or breast-feeding women, smokeless tobacco users, individuals with serious medical conditions—such as a history of cardiovascular disease, uncontrolled hypertension, diabetes, seizure disorders, eating disorders, or psychiatric illness. It is strongly recommended to consult with your physician prior to use. NRT is also questioned for use in conjunction with taking birth control or consuming alcohol.

"Mothers who use snuff or other nicotine replacement therapies may be getting more nicotine than they would if they were smoking cigarettes," says Ana Krieger, MD, Director of the Center for Sleep Medicine at New York Presbyterian Hospital/ Weill Cornell New York City.

It is always a good idea to check in with reputable sources or with a pharmacist or physician before you try out a new product, especially when you are pregnant.

Q#8 "WILL I ALWAYS BE ADDICTED TO NICOTINE?"

As soon as you put out a cigarette you are on your way to breaking the addiction cycle. If you never light up again, you will find your way free of nicotine addiction. It is that straightforward.

Nicotine is an addictive drug. Seeing it as an external force that wants to control your brain and invade your body can help you to push it away. Once you have escaped its clutches, the next step is to make sure you never allow it back into your life ever again.

Remind yourself regularly that you have a new way of living without tobacco products, a strengthened ability to use the word "no" when confronted by practices that don't fit your life as a parent. Understanding addiction and knowing that as little as one puff of one cigarette could hook you back in is important in preventing you from sliding back into behaviours.

Any thoughts or feelings about needing or wanting a cigarette will also pass—unless you nurture them or decide to cave in to them. Over time, the psychological addiction will dissipate if you no longer believe using these products holds any value.

It is possible to get to a place in time where you cannot imagine lighting up a cigarette.

Nicotine addiction-dependency.

Once you have the drug nicotine in your system you will call out for more on a precise schedule. Addiction is the cycle of use and withdrawal. The relief experienced from taking another dose of nicotine is the experience of drug addiction.

If you have ever gone longer than 30 minutes without using the drug nicotine, you will have experienced withdrawal.

If you hear yourself buying into the idea that because nicotine is an addiction you will never be free, then consider seeing it as a dependency. Use whatever word you think will give you the leverage to get yourself off this drug. You can also see it as a relationship that has turned sour and needs to end—like yesterday.

An idea to try on your quit date: How about ending this once and for all in grand style? Look at a cigarette, hold it up to your face, and declare bravely, "This relationship is over."

Throw it in the toilet and, with a grand gesture, flush. It's a fitting end to a nasty product, would you not agree? Select a breakup song for quitting and play it to remind yourself of your achievement in ending your relationship with tobacco products. Two good breakup songs are Taylor Swift's *We Are Never, Ever Getting Back Together* and John Legend's *This Time*.

Q#9 "IS CUTTING DOWN A GOOD STRATEGY FOR QUITTING?"

Some people do succeed by cutting down and it is certainly one component of the Five "D's" strategy discussed on page 48. However, consider the following before you decide to use this method. Giving up smoking completely might be easier than cutting back if cutting back requires an enormous expenditure of energy to stay on a schedule or uses up vast amounts of self-control. Abstaining could make things a lot easier than just a few smokes from time to time.

Remember, as long as there is any nicotine in your life you will be susceptible to its demands. You decide. You are, after all, the expert on you.

Nicotine is not only an addictive drug, it is the *most addictive* of all drugs due to the speed at which it enters the brain—that is, approximately 7 to 10 seconds. It takes as little as one cigarette to wire the brain for addiction, and can take as long as 5 to 10 years for brain cells to return to normal after long-term reliance on tobacco products.

Some individuals will show evidence of addiction within a few days of their first cigarette.

Exercise #4: Using wisdom wisely.

Make a list of any ideas and thoughts that you think may no longer fit with your lifestyle. Prepare to replace them with new and brilliant bits of wisdom that will bring you closer to what you want out of life. Wisdom, ideas, and beliefs should be treated like shoes. If they no longer fit, pick out a new pair. We use thousands of sayings, idioms, metaphors, and beliefs to guide us through our daily lives and every once in awhile it is a good idea to test their validity.

Examples:

- Moderation in all things. (Maybe not if it means a puff of a cigarette will drag you back to the regular use of tobacco products.)
- Absence makes the heart grow fonder. (Maybe not if you find a new and better way to live your life and enjoy the benefits of abstinence.)
- Out of sight out of mind. (Why tempt temptation?)
- Feelings fade unless stimulated. (It will be surprising how quickly you forget all about smoking once you have thrown away the last pack.)
- Nothing ventured, nothing gained. (You will never know unless you try.)

Continue to observe conventional words of wisdom that you frequently use. Decide if the ideas behind the words help or hinder your decisions.

Q#10 "SMOKING HELPS ME HANDLE STRESS. WHAT WILL HAPPEN WHEN I QUIT?"

By responding to stressors in new ways other than smoking you may be undoing years of established behavior patterns, so be gentle with yourself. Think of new and constructive ways to handle stressful situations rather than lighting up or taking a "smoke-break."

Stress is one of the major reasons people give for continuing to smoke or for slipping back to using tobacco products after they have quit. Increased stress, good or bad, is part and parcel of learning new skills and taking on new activities. Parenthood is right up there on many people's lists of top stressors. Preparing for what stressors may be thrown your way is a great strategy when you are planning to quit tobacco products, as is getting to know your own stress-overload warning signs. Preparation can help you head off stress before it shows up and derails your carefully laid-out plans for quitting.

Exercise #5: What could you do during these situations that does not involve smoking?
- A tough day ahead with little sleep.
- A confrontation at work.
- A disagreement with a family member.

Try these suggestions when you feel yourself being pulled off course by stress.
- Take a break and leave the situation to consider your options.
- Call someone and get some help with a situation that's causing you problems.

- Take deep breaths in and then exhale completely, letting it all go.
- Go for a walk or engage in non-task-oriented activities, such as having a bath, to give your brain a break.
- Do gentle exercise. This will help with the release of endorphins.
- Get some rest.
- Put the problem into perspective.
- Resist the urge to please everyone all the time.
- Allow people to solve their own problems in their own time.
- Use your imagination.
- Ask questions and get clarification.
- Remind yourself that not every situation is within your control. You have control over how you respond to a situation and what you decide to do about it, and that's about it.
- Take a five-minute vacation. Close your eyes then take in a deep, slow breath and then breathe out equally slowly. Imagine yourself in a beautiful place, taking some time to create a space in your imagination—a beach, a castle, a forest, a meadow, or a pool in which you are floating. Choose a place that is safe for you. Visualize it as much as you can and bring color to it. Imagine a green forest, turquoise waters, or blue skies. Slowly open your eyes, refreshed.

A conditioned response is doing things in the old, familiar way. Ideas to try for changing patterns of behavior when stressed:

- If you don't usually talk it out, try to do just that.
- Resist rehashing the same old stuff in the same way with the same people. Feelings fade unless they are stimulated and bringing up all the old stuff may just make you feel worse.

- If you usually step in, try stepping back.
- Do something different.
- Tell yourself no one is perfect and brush yourself off.
- Get a good night's sleep and come at the stressful issue or event tomorrow.
- Count to 10.
- If you are really stressed, put your hands over your head. This makes breathing easier as it opens up your chest muscles and your rib cage.
- Sit down, or lie down, and bring yourself into this moment in time. Let the past and future go for now.
- Allow yourself to daydream. Studies show that during 50% of our waking hours our minds are wandering. Let your mind wander to pleasant lands.
- Find any way to laugh or to entertain yourself.
- When we are stressed, the body responds by focusing on the supply of energy to the muscles so you can fight or flee. This is not the time to deal with mind-challenging pursuits or to further deplete your energy with goal-oriented tasks.
- Go for a pleasant walk in a safe place with someone whose company you enjoy.

Exercise #6: The experience of smoking.
1. Do you smoke when you are:
Angry Happy Anxious Bored Tired Hungry Relaxed Stressed Frightened?
Circle any words that apply to your experiences.

2. Fill in your answer to the missing word here:
When you are _____, you drink water.

Complete this sentence:

When you are stressed you _____

When you are hungry, you eat. When you are tired, you sleep. If you smoke because you are feeling stressed, then one thing you know for sure is that you are experiencing stress, and you need to pay attention to what is causing you stress. Try to keep the two things separate. When you are stressed you are stressed, and when you are smoking you are smoking.

Smoking creates physical stress, which activates the central nervous system. It creates its own problems and does not address stress in a productive way.

A question for you:

Is continuing to smoke during pregnancy causing you stress?

If you answered yes, then it is a time to accept a new belief: Smoking tobacco products *creates* stress.

Practice non-doing more often.

- Nap or take a break with your feet up.
- Meditate or do gentle stretching.
- Focus on your breath.
- Get out into nature every day.
- Listen to music.
- Practice mindfulness. For example, when you are having a shower, use all your senses to stay with the experience. Keep drawing your attention back to the moment, the experience, at hand.

Handling stress in your communications.

Pay particular attention to how you communicate in a stressful situation. See if you can make any changes to reduce any stress in your relationships at work or at home. Try out new ways to handle difficult problems and situations.

Keep the desired outcome front and center in your mind. Recall how you dealt with this or a similar situation before and remember the outcome. If you want to change the outcome, change your approach. If what you have been doing has not been working, it is time for a new plan. With a little creativity you might be surprised at how many options are available. Sometimes a letter will work better than a conversation and sometimes a conversation is the only way to go. Be realistic and realize that change may not happen overnight.

Recognize what causes you stress.

One of the most important things you can do to reduce the amount of stress in your life is to recognize when you have simply had enough and need to rest or step away. The HALT strategy is a very effective tool for realizing when you are susceptible to the effects of stress. HALT stands for: too hungry, too angry, too lonely, or too tired. Any one of these four factors can add to your stress levels. Know your limits and do your best to avoid overburdening yourself. This will help make you less susceptible to stress and to going back to your old ways of reacting.

The best antidote to stress.

Our best antidote to stress is always with us—our ability to breathe. When you balance your breathing, a sense of calm will flood over both your physiological and your psychological being and things will be set right, including your ability to think clearly and make good decisions on a course of action that is in your best interests. One definition of the word "courage" is that precise moment in time when you choose to replace the rapid breathing activated by the fight or flight (also known as fight or flee) stress response with normal breathing.

On average, North Americans experience 60 to 90 stress episodes a day. Each time this happens, the parasympathetic nervous system and normal breathing patterns are disrupted. Stress also activates the central nervous system, which results in shallow and faster breathing, a racing heart, and blood flowing from the major organs, including the brain, to the extremities to enable the fight or flight response.

Understanding the basics of breathing is one of the most important aspects of handling stress. (Bonus: it can also help you prepare for labor.) There are four parts to the breathing process:

1. Inhalation.
2. Pause. The moment at the end of inhalation before the beginning of exhalation. Holding at "pause" can create a feeling of pressure, anxiety, and is generally stress producing.
3. Exhalation.
4. Surrender. The moment at the end of exhalation right before the next inhalation. This is the moment of letting it all go. It is recommended that you linger here to enjoy a feeling of deep relaxation and release. Breathe again when you feel the urge to do so.

Exercise #7: Attention to breathing.
Sit with your feet parallel to one another. Close your eyes. Put your hands on your throat and breathe in through your nose. Now move your hands to your belly and experience the end

of inhalation. Now, with little pause, place your hands on your heart and let the breath begin to leave your body. When the exhalation is over, place your hands on your throat and deepen the feeling of letting go. Some people like to place their hands on their face for the exhalation. Repeat this as many times as you like, but do not count as this will prevent you from relaxing and will keep you in a busy state of mind.

You can learn a great deal about the state of your emotional world by paying attention to your breath. Did you know that when you are sad and depressed your exhalation will be prolonged, and when you are angry your exhalation will quicken?

By taking a few minutes to balance your breath or pay attention to your breath, you can influence how you are feeling and increase your ability to handle stress.

Naturally relaxed breathing is nostril breathing. Breathing through your mouth on a continuous basis will contribute to anxiety. Breathing through your nose, however, is calming. When you breathe through your nose you will automatically smile, which is a wonderful way to approach life. If you are interested in learning more about breath and breathing, you might want to explore the splendid world of yoga, mindfulness, and meditation.

Q#11 "I KNOW ABOUT THE RISKS, BUT I CAN'T GET THROUGH A DAY WITHOUT LIGHTING UP. HOW DO OTHER PREGNANT WOMEN FIND IT SO EASY?"

Although many women quit when they learn they are pregnant, many of them return to using tobacco products after the baby is born. By taking the time now to thoroughly explore why you are continuing to smoke, you actually have an advantage over many of those people who seem to have found quitting "easy." By seriously challenging your perception of your relationship with tobacco products you stand a good chance not only of quitting but also of achieving lasting success.

Q#12 "IS IT TRUE THAT NICOTINE IS THE HARDEST DRUG TO GET OFF?"

Once you were hooked on nicotine you were handed another limiting belief that served to further entrench you as a regular tobacco-product consumer.

It is nearly impossible to have a discussion about quitting smoking with a group of people without someone bringing up the idea that quitting smoking is difficult. People often voluntarily add that it is not only hard, but, in fact, is also "one of the most difficult if not the hardest things a human being can ever attempt."

A basic principal in marketing is to tell stories about a given product that will be easy for customers to buy into. It was simple to get people who smoke to believe that it was hard to stop smoking—it offered a way out of quitting.

At first glance it may appear empathetic or even sympathetic when friends and acquaintances talk about how hard it is to quit smoking, but telling someone how incredibly hard quitting is going to be is not helpful, especially when it is not accurate.

The people who work for the industry must love it.

From this point on there is no need to ever use the word "hard" again in a conversation about quitting. Quitting is just quitting.

Statistics about quitting smoking.

1. Over 90% of the estimated 37 million people who quit in the first 20 years after the U.S. Surgeon General's Report linked the use of tobacco products to cancer did so unaided.
2. In a fascinating study of ex-smokers in the 1980s, 53% of ex-smokers said it was "not at all difficult to stop," 27% said "it was fairly difficult," and the remaining 20% said they had "found it very difficult."
3. From the 1970s onward, smoking prevalence in North America fell rapidly until the mid-1990s. From the 1990s onward, the rates of decline slowed and from 2007 to the present there has been little change.

What we choose to believe.

We choose what we believe and sometimes we mistakenly buy into the wrong ideas. In an article in a 2012 edition of *Best Health* magazine, a journalist compared contradictory results from research about alcohol consumption. The subtitle read, "Nearly 80% of people over the age of 18 drink alcohol regularly so it's crucial to know what to believe." This article demonstrated how increasingly difficult it is to know who and what to believe in our crowded world of news reports and countless studies.

The article noted:

Alcohol increases your cancer risk. Alcohol decreases your cancer risk. It harms your brain. It helps your brain. It stresses you out. It relaxes you. It harms your bones. It helps your bones. It causes weight gain. It helps you stay thin. It will kill you. It will help you live longer.

In the same publication, another article quoted Dr. David Spence, of the London, Ontario, Health Sciences Centre University Hospital: "In August of 2012 a study found regular consumption of egg yolks to be about two-thirds as bad as smoking for increasing build-up of carotid plaque."

Whether or not this statement is accurate, the potential influence that such public announcements can have on what we decide to buy and consume is significant. In our fast-paced world we take bits of information from a multitude of sources and do the best we can to get on with our lives without creating too much damage.

Dr. Serge Renaud studied the effects of alcohol on health for over 40 years as the Director of Cardiology at the French National Institute of Health and Medical Research. He appeared on the television show *60 Minutes* in 1991 to an audience of 33 million people and reported that alcohol, specifically red wine, could reduce the risks of heart disease. In the month following the program, sales of red wine increased by 2.5 million bottles in the United States. The show was repeated in 1992 and the sale of red wine went up by 49% for that month. The doctor also called for a total prohibition on binge drinking and suggested that the amount of alcohol that could prove beneficial was so small that one merely needed a sniff. The relevancy of quantity had been lost in the excitement of it all. Sometimes we get it wrong.

Q#13 "DOES SMOKING HELP WITH WEIGHT LOSS?"

Most unfortunately, the idea that nicotine suppresses appetite or contributes to weight loss is now widely accepted and may have contributed to young women's increasing uptake of tobacco products. Many things can calm your appetite without risking your health: drinking a glass of water, getting adequate fiber, and eating a well-balanced, healthy meal. Associating nicotine with dieting is not useful. It is a limiting belief that works against your best interests.

➤ PEOPLE WHO SMOKE ARE AS PRONE TO OBESITY AS NON-SMOKERS IF THEY OVEREAT REGULARLY, DO NOT EXERCISE, SUFFER FROM CHRONIC STRESS, OR DO NOT GET ENOUGH SLEEP.

Having a healthy appetite and enjoying the satisfaction food can provide is one of the basic human pleasures. If you attempt to suppress your appetite, the feeling of hunger becomes more difficult to differentiate from other sensations and a pattern of eating for reasons other than hunger can emerge.

Ditch the diet, ditch the appetite-suppressant idea, and identify and savor your feelings—each and every one of them, including natural hunger. Suppressing your appetite with nicotine or tobacco is a tired idea, as is the idea that we all need to strive to be model thin.

Carine Roitfeld, former editor of French *Vogue*, wrote in 2011,

Now I decide I will never use a cigarette again in any shoot. When you're doing fashion pictures, you're talking to lots of figures; some are very young, and they're like sponges. So if your girl is smoking a cigarette, they can say, Oh, my God, it's smart to smoke a cigarette, it's good for the look, so I'm going to have one, too. And it's totally stupid. It's an easy solution to make a picture more interesting, but it's not the only solution. And now it's like, forgive me for all these cigarettes I've put in all these issues.

A major concern for many people considering quitting smoking is that they will gain weight. Some people do gain weight when they quit, but only because they use food to replace smoking—not because of some dramatic metabolic change or the lack of nicotine in their system. Eating is eating and smoking is smoking. If you put anything in your mouth to prevent food passing your lips, you will influence your weight. There is nothing magical about the connection between tobacco products and weight management.

Studies suggest that the best way to maintain a healthy weight is to never go on a diet, to write down what you eat, to not forbid yourself anything in particular unless there is a medical reason, to keep an eye on balance and quantities, and to weigh yourself regularly. Other experts suggest that you should just stick to what you like and watch your portion sizes. After all, three mouthfuls of anything never made anyone fat.

One additional point worth mentioning is that currently, on average, Americans get close to 30% of their daily calories from products devoid of any nutrients. The empty-calories culprits are alcohol, sugary drinks, and sweets. Now that you are pregnant you will want to eliminate all alcohol and look at replacing those calories saved with good, nutrient-rich foods that will benefit you and your growing baby.

If you are particularly concerned about the issue of weight gain and quitting smoking, pay extra attention to any feelings of temptation or deprivation. One of the best strategies for dealing with these particular feelings is to remind yourself that this is drug addiction and the drug is messing with you. It wants back in. Remind yourself that by quitting tobacco, you and your baby will have a healthier life together.

Who are they kidding?
In 1968 the Virginia Slims cigarette line was launched as a strategy to attract a broader female market. The industry's target market was young women, aged 18 to 35, who were fashion conscious, desirous of being thin, and predominately liberal-minded. The promotional campaigns for the Slims fit right in with themes involving women's emancipation, and the ads frequently featured fashion models.

Virginia Slims are still on the market but at least the derogatory slogans of the last century have been retired.

You've come a long way, baby
To get where you've got to today
You've got your own cigarette now, baby
You've come a long, long way.

The tobacco industry has used its vast wealth to hire the best market manipulators on the planet and the creativity that has gone into the tobacco campaigns over the past 60 years has been nothing short of brilliant. It is, however, tragic that such talent was squandered on having people develop an unhealthy dependency that can lead to disease and death.

What else does the tobacco industry talk you into believing?
A tobacco print ad appeared in a 2009 publication of American *Vogue* for Davidoff cigarettes. The woman in the photograph is in her early 20s. She is thin, with gleaming teeth and gorgeous flowing hair. She is sitting in a bar with a cocktail in front of her. The text reads:

Luxury Takes a New Shape.

You're discerning in everything you do. It's all part of the graceful style that you have created. And the sophisticated details of Davidoff Slims cigarettes are a perfect complement to your elegant profile. LIFE IS RICH: Davidoff Cigarettes.

Marketers will continue to do what they do best, but we do not have to buy into any of their ideas or the industry's propaganda.

The Tobacco Master Settlement Agreement.

The Tobacco Master Settlement Agreement (MSA) was signed in 1998 by the four largest American tobacco companies and the attorneys general of 46 states. The tobacco industry was forced to compensate the nation for a portion of the healthcare costs associated with caring for people with smoking-related diseases. The amount was to be paid over a 25-year period and amounted to more than $240 billion.

Under the MSA, the tobacco industry was also forced to stop certain tobacco marketing practices, including the use of cartoon characters in the promotion of their products. It was established not only that young children were attracted to the images of Joe Camel, but also that this primed children for tobacco use in their youth.

How did the industry respond to the weighty penalties placed on them for being found guilty of invoked damages on the public's health?

According to Harvard School of Public Health research published in 2007, the amount of nicotine that smokers consumed per cigarette, regardless of brand or manufacturer, increased an average of 1.6% per year from 1998 to 2004. The Harvard study claims that cigarette manufacturers have intentionally increased their products' nicotine levels to produce a more addictive product. The research found that nicotine levels in cigarettes from all major manufacturers increased by 11% between 1997 and 2005. The tobacco industry dismissed these findings outright.

The MSA, for all intents and purposes, was principally a new excise tax on cigarettes. Following the agreement, the four principal tobacco companies—Philip Morris, R.J. Reynolds, Brown and Williamson, and Lorillard—raised their prices more than 45 cents per pack. The costs of the settlement, as predicted, were passed on to consumers. (Allan M. Brandt, *The Cigarette Century: The Rise, Fall and Deadly Persistence of the Product that Defined America.*)

In 2013 Imperial Tobacco introduced a new line of cigarettes. It hired prominent artists from around the world to make every detail an inspiring piece of art and turn a habitual cigarette package into a unique masterpiece of contemporary art.

In 2012 the Australian government implemented a public policy for all tobacco products to be sold in olive-colored, plain packaging that featured graphic health warnings. The tobacco industry claims it will challenge the plain packaging policy in the courts.

On May 31, 2011, Central Park in New York City went smoke-free. Camel retaliated with full-page color ads in publications including *USA Today* that read:

NYC Smokers enjoy freedom without the flame. Smokers, switch to Camel SNUS and reclaim the world's greatest city. No matter where you go, or what you do, Camel

SNUS is the perfect tobacco pleasure to enjoy virtually anywhere. Camel SNUS—the pleasure's all yours.

The upper right-hand corner features the Camel logo and the slogan BREAK FREE. In small type to the left is the following industry-generated wording: "Share your support for tobacco freedom at CamelSNUS.com/solution."

A full-page color ad ran the banner message: "NYC SMOKERS RISE ABOVE THE BAN."

The bottom of the page ran a warning in black and white: "WARNING: This product can cause gum disease and tooth loss."

It is disturbing to look back at the messages coming out of the marketing machine of the tobacco industry from the early 20th century onward. We now know that the tobacco industry knew well in advance of public announcements in 1964 about the significant health risks associated with using their products. They continued to push out advertising campaigns promoting the idea of freedom even though they knew the risks they were exposing their customers to.

An ad for Tipalet cigarettes from the 1970s depicts a woman gazing longingly at a man who is holding a Tipalet. The caption reads: "Blow in her face and she'll follow you anywhere."

The text of the ad reads:

Hit her with tangy Tipalet Cherry. Or rich, grape-y Tipalet Burgundy. Or luscious Tipalet Blueberry. It's Wild! Tipalet. ... A puff in her direction and she'll follow you, anywhere. Oh yes ... you get smoking satisfaction without inhaling smoke. Smokers of America do yourself a flavor. Make your next cigarette a Tipalet.

Equally reprehensible were the industry's efforts to taint agencies, and/or individuals, who were outspoken about the industry's tactics by suggesting that their critics were akin to prohibitionists and posed a threat to an individual's rights and freedoms. The most effective tobacco-prevention strategies have come from the organizations and individuals who dared to take a stand against Big Tobacco and who demanded new legislation to better protect the public's health.

The tobacco industry has continued to produce products that will end up costing half the people who use them on a long-term basis an average of 12 years of life, with millions more harmed by exposure to second- and third-hand smoke.

Why has the tobacco industry escaped serious scrutiny? Because the tobacco epidemic and the public health issues that are at its core have not generated sufficient salience. Salience in this context is that mix of ingredients, topicality and urgency, that forces tobacco issues to the top of the political agenda and holds them there. There is a public health strategy to help reverse this tobacco normalization process. It is called tobacco industry de-normalization or TID. This strategy plays hardball with the people who are after our kids. The cigarette manufacturers loathe this strategy, because it strikes at the core of their business, dishonestly obtained normalcy. (Garfield Mahood, when acting as Executive Director, Non-Smokers' Rights Association, Canada.)

Note: Carine Roitfeld includes cigarettes in an editorial for the March 2013 issue of CR Fashion.

Q#14 "SMOKING HELPS ME GO TO SLEEP AT NIGHT. NOW I AM PREGNANT BUT I HAVEN'T DECIDED IF I AM GOING TO QUIT OR NOT. I LIKE IT."

Nicotine is a known stimulant and when used before bedtime, it actually interrupts sleep patterns and has been linked to sleep disorders. It is always best to check to make sure that beliefs about tobacco are accurate and that your strategies are working in your best interests. Many people all over the world have trouble sleeping from time to time, but taking up smoking is not a recommended solution. If a friend approached you about insomnia, would you recommend she start to smoke?

The following story may put this in perspective.

A man who was worried about his dogs getting fleas started sprinkling seasoning powder over their food as he had read that garlic repelled fleas. After the man had been doing this for quite some time, both his dogs got very sick and then died. It was suspected that they had developed a blood disorder as a result of eating the seasoning powder that contained onions and garlic, both of which are dangerous food ingredients that cause sickness in dogs, cats, and livestock.

Start to notice the things you tell yourself. Take a second look and determine if these beliefs are helping you or holding you back.

Exercise #8: Consider your response to the following ideas.
- Do you believe you are addicted to nicotine or do you believe it is a habit?
- Do you believe that habits are hard to break and that it takes 21 days to do so?

Habits, such as sleeping on one particular side of the bed, walking the same way to work each day, or brushing our teeth in the morning, are not necessarily hard to break. When given new data we can and do change our habits. We find a new way to cross the street if something is blocking our regular route. Habits are harder to break if you believe they are hard to break.

Name a dessert you like to eat. How often do you eat it? How often do you use tobacco products?

Desserts are wonderful, but do you eat them every 45 minutes, or every couple of hours, or 20 times a day?

Eating dessert regularly is a habit. Smoking a cigarette every 45 minutes is an addiction. Addictive substances have your number on speed dial. This is the difference between a habit and an addiction-dependency.

Tips for a good night's sleep.
Choose a few of these ideas to try:
- Darken the room as much as possible.
- Aim to go to bed at the same time each night.
- Keep the room cool and well ventilated.
- Aim to never go to bed mad. Let it all go for now.
- Practice yoga to reduce your physical and psychological stress of the day.
- Have a warm bath before bed.
- Keep pets off the bed.
- Create a bedtime routine.

Q#15 "I KNOW WOMEN WHO USE MARIJUANA WHEN THEY ARE PREGNANT AND MY FRIEND TOLD ME IT WOULD HELP WITH MORNING SICKNESS. WHAT DO YOU THINK?"

The reason marijuana cannot be recommended, besides still being labeled an illicit drug, is because the limited research results we have show evidence of serious risks associated with using marijuana during pregnancy. There are other ways to handle morning sickness, and marijuana cannot be recommended at any time during pregnancy.

Between 50% and 80% of women will experience some degree of morning sickness during their pregnancy. For a small percentage of women, morning sickness has the potential to become a very serious health threat. In some circumstances, morning sickness medications may be prescribed. In that case, their possible side effects will be explained. If you are ever unclear about something that you have been recommended to take, ask a healthcare professional. If you still are unsure, ask again.

An additional note: As with alcohol, if marijuana is given extra powers through a belief that it will take away your problems or can be relied on to have a specific effect, it can cause you serious problems. If you need help to deal with drug dependency you can contact the National Council on Alcohol and Drug Dependence on 1-800-622-2255.

Q#16 "I FEEL LIKE A CIGARETTE. NOW WHAT DO I DO?"

We do not need to respond to or act on every feeling we have. You can think about smoking or feel like a cigarette and still not smoke. We can be frightened and not freak out.

If you choose to smoke, recognize it as your choice to make but keep working on ways to uncover why you are continuing to smoke. There are likely reasons why you are smoking, other than the fact that nicotine is an addictive drug and you "wanted a cig."

It is always frightening when you attempt something for the first time and you find yourself out on a limb. What you choose to do out there on that limb is what makes all the difference.

Forget quitting for the moment and consider another scenario.

If you set out a plan to go for a walk every day because it is good for your mental health, how long do you think it would be before you started feeling resistant to the new plan and you stopped doing what you set out to do?

Set out to walk every day around the block and notice when you start to feel some resistance to going for a walk. Walk anyway. Write down any time you notice resistance or experience feelings of annoyance at having to follow through on your plan to walk. It could be that the issue is not the problem of deciding to quit smoking but rather your response or reaction to feelings of resistance. Experiment with a few more habits, such as flossing your teeth every day or drinking water regularly throughout the day, and note what levels of resistance show up.

Chalk up your feelings of resistance to your rebellious nature and decide to find rebellions worth fighting—like fighting the urge to buy another pack of cigarettes.

Notice how you talk to yourself. Watch for clues about how your feelings are controlling what you do and how they may be preventing you from following through on your carefully thought-out plans designed to get you what you really want in life.

Instead of saying to yourself:

"I feel like having a cigarette" or "I don't feel like going for a walk."

Say to yourself:

"I feel like having a cigarette but I am not going to have one. I am not going respond to every strong feeling that comes along."

Tell yourself:

"I don't feel like walking today. It's raining but I am going to walk, because I have made a promise to myself and I know that I will feel better after I do. I will bring my grumpy self along and go for a walk. It will only take 10 minutes and that is what I have decided to do."

Q#17 "HOW DO I HANDLE GOING OUT WITH MY FRIENDS AND NOT LIGHTING UP AGAIN? WHAT WILL HAPPEN WHEN I START DRINKING AGAIN?"

Sometimes smoking cessation programs recommend that you clear out the drawers of all smoking products or reminders. Why tempt temptation? The best policy is out of sight and out of mind. If it helps to clean out the drawers and your pockets then by all means do so.

However, do not lull yourself into a false sense of security by making your house a clean zone or deciding who you will stay in contact with once you quit. You have control over what you choose to do. When your beliefs are aligned with doing things in your best interests, you need not fear being tempted by the sight or smell of products that no longer have an appeal for you.

There is a world of difference between doing what you feel like doing and doing what needs to be done. Our feelings are our feelings and our actions are our actions. The ability to coexist with difficult feelings or thoughts and get on with what needs to be done is the basis of self-control. When we can allow feelings and thoughts to exist while we get on with what we need to do in our lives, we become free to feel and think fully.

You see yourself as a free spirit and pride yourself on your spontaneous nature. If you feel a sense of resistance welling up in response to the idea of having to plan ahead and create a quit plan, you need to look at the bigger picture and remember what is most important to you right now.

Self-control and self-discipline will get you what you most want out of life. Real freedom is not having a constant and relentless problem interrupting your life. It is about taking back your personal power to effect change and define your creative and spontaneous life on your terms.

"Freedom is the ability to live your life fully and meaningfully regardless of the range of feelings which occupy your mind and heart at any given moment." —Gregg Krech

Q#18 "I COULDN'T QUIT FOR THE REASON OF PROTECTING MY OWN HEALTH. IS LOW SELF-ESTEEM WHY I CAN'T QUIT?"

It is possible that you are speaking to yourself in a derogatory way, but does this really happen every time you light up? Is this really the reason for continuing to smoke?

We know that nicotine will regularly call your name and that it has its own schedule, but it is too convenient to draw the conclusion that your smoking is linked to low self-esteem and that your negative thoughts keep time with nicotine's demanding schedule. If a person smokes regularly, cigarettes will call out to them every 30 to 45 minutes. However, people do not suffer thoughts of self-loathing in such an organized fashion. There are simply too many things to attend to and we cannot be harboring thoughts that dampen our self-esteem all day long.

To stop torturing yourself—and to move on with your plan to quit smoking—you need to let go of the belief that lack of self-esteem is preventing you from quitting. In fact, it is not a lack of self-esteem but too much self-esteem that can most hinder an attempt to quit. Studies show that an overly self-assured individual may take risks because they believe they are strong enough to cope with the consequences.

Q#19 "WHAT CAN I DO TO IMPROVE MY CHANCES OF SUCCESS? I DON'T WANT TO WASTE ANY TIME NOW THAT I KNOW I AM PREGNANT."

Now is a good time to work on your quit plan. Remember that you will have a better chance of succeeding if you prepare for specific situations in which you may have the urge to smoke. The best offense is a good defense. Defensively, you can prepare for the urges you may experience by listing your triggers or situations when you would normally use tobacco products, and deciding ahead of time what you will do instead. Make a list in your quit plan of the positive steps you will take when you have an urge to smoke. These steps will keep you in control of your life. A cigarette won't. For example, if you have an urge to smoke after a lengthy meal, a good alternative would be to get up and take a walk, brush your teeth, or have a shower. You only need a three-minute activity to get you over this hurdle. There is no need for elaborate schemes or expensive options. A spa day is certainly nice, but it is not a very realistic or practical trigger-counter defense.

Know your triggers and danger zones.
Identify what might come up that could take you off course, and think of other things to do. For example:
- If you are feeling grumpy, go for a walk, rest, or play music for the baby and you to enjoy.
- If you are hungry, have a piece of fruit or a glass of water or prepare a meal.
- If you have a headache, sit down and put a cold cloth on your neck, ask for a massage from someone, or have a warm bath or shower. You could also close your eyes and rest without stimuli such as television, turn off your computer and take a break with your feet up, or try gentle acupuncture by pressing the flesh between your thumb and first finger and breathing deeply.
- If you are restless, go for a walk or read a book or magazine.
- If you are having trouble sleeping, read, or get up and have a glass of cold milk, possibly with a small bowl of cereal.
- If you are anxious, focus on your breathing.
- If you are feeling bored or lonely, contact a friend.
- If you are angry or upset, think about what you want to happen or change, or take a break and regroup.

Preparing for a tobacco-free life.
The following suggestions are practical ways to work through urges that could possibly challenge your resolve to accomplish what you have set out to do.

Change how you think about tobacco products.

When you have the urge to smoke, say these statements to yourself:

- "Smoking is not the only way to deal with my problems. Actually, smoking is making many things in my life worse not better. It is taking my time and money and risking my health. It is interfering with my relationships and making me feel ashamed and just plain awful."
- "The benefits of quitting now are huge. I am in control."
- "It only costs the tobacco industry about 5 cents to make a pack of cigarettes. I don't want to give them any more of my hard-earned money. I need it for more important things."
- "I am now in much better control of my future health."

Change what you do.

When you have the urge to smoke, try one of these activities instead:

- Read your quit plan. Remember what is most important to you: having a healthy lifestyle to support your family and yourself.
- Read a book, listen to music, or watch a favorite show.
- Focus on preparing to be a parent, read parenting materials, and plan ahead.
- If you are having doubts about your ability to quit smoking, remember all the possibilities.

Possibilities

It is possible to beat the statistics

It is also possible to better your chances

It is possible to accelerate the average time to quit
It is possible to defy all of the studies
It is possible to win
It is possible to ask for some help
It is possible for you to live a life free of products
That are causing you distress, burdening your health
And your relationships

Q#20 "WHEN I QUIT, FOR HOW LONG WILL THE CRAVINGS CONTINUE?"

Studies conducted in 2009 by the National Institute of Drug Abuse reported that nicotine-dependent people who had smoked one pack a day for an average of 21 years demonstrated that, after 6 to 12 weeks of abstinence, their brain receptor levels were the same as those of non-smokers. Others studies suggest that the time required may be significantly greater.

When you read the paragraph above, did you jump to the conclusion that you would have to suffer through months or years of awful withdrawal symptoms or constant urges?

Why do you think that might have happened? As long as you view quitting as something that could create discomfort, part of your mind will be looking for ways to escape and get you off the hook. It is important to remember that you can get through withdrawal. The experience is quite different for everyone.

It is even more important that you remind yourself that you have experienced withdrawal before. You have lived in withdrawal for the entire time you have been smoking. That is the experience of addiction. Every two hours the amount of nicotine in your body declines by half, so it does not take very long to be physically clean of this drug. After a night's sleep you wake up in a physical state of withdrawal. This happens any time you go without a regular dose of nicotine.

It is possible to quit smoking without ever getting into the intricate details of brain chemistry, dopamine pathways, and nicotine receptors. Some people find it very helpful to know about and understand these processes, but for other people it makes little, if any, difference.

Reminder: Take care not to underestimate how much your expectations, which are created by your imagination, can influence outcomes.

Exercise #9: *What do you know about the experience of withdrawal?*

Reflect on the following questions:

1. What is your experience when you open your eyes first thing in the morning?
2. How desperate are you in the morning for a first cigarette?
3. What do you already know about the experience of withdrawal and urges?
4. How bad have withdrawal symptoms been for you?

On average, a craving or urge to smoke in the first few days of quitting lasts for three minutes, the time it takes to boil an egg. These urges have a beginning, middle, and an end—similar to a contraction in childbirth.

Tips for dealing with urge to smoke.

- Sit down.
- Lie down.

- Think about something else. We can only have one thought at a time so one strategy is to distract your thoughts of smoking by simply thinking something else: sing a song, recite a poem, read something, read anything. Distractions give you something else to do when you feel the urge to smoke.
- Sip eight ounces of water.
- Carry a piece of fruit with you to eat when you feel the urge to smoke. Dried fruit travels especially well.
- Write out a list of effective constructive distractions you can use as needed. Be as specific as possible.
- Find ways to stimulate the release of endorphins. Endorphins, one of the brain's feel-good chemicals and the body's natural painkiller, may be stimulated and released in the body by the following: listening to music, walking in nature, exercising, laughing, being tickled, gentle touching, consuming spicy food, smelling vanilla and lavender, and enjoying both deep relaxation and its opposite—excitement. Endorphins can help with quitting smoking by creating pleasant feelings and improving your mood.
- Repeat a strategy or tip that works. Repeating a pattern is one of the tools recommended in early labor to build confidence. It is especially helpful when the presenting experiences are new and unfamiliar.

Q#21 "DO STRATEGIES AND DISTRACTIONS WORK?"
Yes, distractions can work to take your mind off the urge to smoke. When you are successful, reward yourself and celebrate the fact that you are tobacco-free.

Celebrate that you have freed yourself from tobacco products. Tell someone that you have quit and ask this person to join your celebration.

Plan to counter an urge with a distraction. You truly can over-power the urge and build on your success.

You could walk around the corner of a building and have smoke blow in your face, or someone could offer you a cigarette. Maybe you'll find yourself at a sales counter and be tempted to buy some cigarettes. This moment when the drug is calling your name is the one you need to prepare for. The last thing you want—or need—is a craving to sideswipe you and take you off course. This is when having a plan is crucial.

You don't want all your efforts to go up in a puff of smoke. It takes only one cigarette to bring the addiction back into your system, creating the whole cycle of dependency all over again. If it does happen and you do slip and have a cigarette, pick your-self up, brush yourself off, continue to believe in your plan, and carry on your good work.

Temporary measures.
Distraction as a strategy to fight off cravings is very helpful, but it is only a temporary measure. Until you address what precisely is holding you to tobacco products, you will need to rely on strategies, tips, and plenty of willpower, motivators, and self-control to stay the course. The permanent solution to not using tobacco products is to dampen the desire to smoke by destroy-ing the idea that they have any value in your current life. By damping down the desire and increasing your ability to exercise willpower and self-control, you stand a great chance at ending this problem once and for all. This doable, double-sided method

can help you get these products out of your life.

Q#22 "WHY IS IT THAT I SOMETIMES FEEL LIKE I HAVE PLENTY OF WILLPOWER AND AT OTHER TIMES I DON'T FEEL LIKE I HAVE ENOUGH TO KEEP ME FROM SMOKING?"

Willpower gives out over time and, like your muscles, it requires rest and replenishment to keep on performing. The more decisions you have to make, the more you have to do to restore your supply of willpower. However, relying on willpower to see you through is not your best strategy when it comes to quitting smoking—or for any other pursuit in which you want to achieve lasting results. Willpower is strongest in the morning. That might get you to an early morning yoga class, but it will not be enough to help you to stay off tobacco products permanently.

To conserve willpower, apply the following tips in the early days of quitting:

- Simplify where you can.
- Aim to make decisions. Deliberating over long periods of time uses up willpower. This is a great reason for setting a quit date and sticking to it.
- If you start to feel tempted or deprived, take a break and do something relaxing: go for a walk, read, listen to music, have a nap, have a small glass of juice or a piece of fruit.
- If you have a big decision to make and are feeling like you are losing control, consider sleeping on it and seeing how you feel first thing in the morning when your willpower is stronger.
- Send someone else to do the shopping if you have just quit.

Delegate as much as you can. This is one way in which someone else can support you in your quit effort. You can ask someone to help with some errands that may tax your willpower without getting into a discussion about quitting.

- Set schedules and routines, such as going to bed at the same time or exercising at the same time each day.
- Remember to make your strategies fit your life. Only use ideas that are realistic for you.
- Relax and listen to music, or enjoy hobbies and pursuits that you enjoy.

The pleasure of doing the same thing, in the same way every day, shouldn't be over looked." —Gretchen Rubin

Tip: Decrease your desire to smoke with the following strategies:
- Review the benefits and rewards of quitting on pages 15–16, 93–95.
- Say "NO" out loud in response to an urge to smoke.
- Take part in the conversation in your head that is trying to lure or trick you back to smoking. Prepare a script so you know what to say.
- Make it more difficult to get to your cigarettes by leaving the pack in your car.
- Make it more difficult to smoke by making it easy to do something else. Place your running shoes at the door so you are ready to go for a walk. Buy yourself an umbrella, an iPod, or anything else that will make the walk enjoyable. With the extra money you will be saving by not smoking you can treat yourself to things that will support your efforts.

Q#23 "SOME OF THE THINGS I HAVE READ SCARE ME. WHERE CAN I GET GOOD INFORMATION THAT WON'T MAKE ME FEEL TERRIBLE?"

Some well-intentioned individuals draw the conclusion that if they provide the reasons for quitting to those who smoke, smokers will automatically take the next step and quit.

In your own experience, does having a strong list of the reasons for quitting help move you ahead or does it serve to entrench you in a position of defensiveness and denial? Does knowing the risks of raising a child who will be around second-hand smoke help or push you back? You get to decide how much information is helpful. Some people find information about the risks helpful and other people find it overwhelming. Do you want to be lectured or nurtured? If you think hard-hitting, stern lectures will scare you into quitting, you can find plenty of them online and in bookstores. This book, however, is grounded in the belief that love beats fear every time.

If 95% of smokers have stated that they wish they could quit and the majority of them are aware of the very good reasons for quitting, would you not agree that we need to look at other ways of helping an individual quit instead of simply telling them about the next proven risk factor? Exactly.

This is why we have included some information on the associated risks connected to smoking, but it is not our primary focus.

If you do find information on the risks helpful, take care what you read, both online and in print. Stick to reputable sources. There is a list of reputable sources at the back of this book and we suggest that you stick to those when looking for answers. The Centers for Disease Control is one of the best places to find information. The World Health Organization and the website of the Surgeon General of the United States are other excellent resources. Your physician or midwife can be good people to turn to for information, understanding, and advice about referral programs.

In addition to reading this book, you might look at other effective tobacco-dependence treatment programs that have been proven to be beneficial, including individual, group, and telephone counseling.

Informed consent.
The majority of people start smoking before they reach adulthood, with some studies suggesting that upward of 25% of regular users of tobacco products started before the age of 10. This means many smokers were customers before the age of legal and informed consent. We have age limits on purchasing tobacco products to give people the opportunity to learn about the full effects these products will likely have on their bodies as well as the impact they will have on other people who will be affected by the second- and third-hand smoke. Collectively, we don't want our kids to start smoking and we make rules, laws, and regulations to that end. Yet, as the initiation rates sadly show, those measures pale in comparison to the tobacco industry's ability to attract new customers. Tobacco industry marketing outspends tobacco prevention dollars by 20:1 or more. The tobacco industry is not going away anytime soon and these companies will continue to capture new markets.

Focus on the fact that in all probability the industry got you into this before you had the opportunity to understand exactly what you were getting involved in. To learn more about the tobacco industry visit www.thetruth.com. Truth is funded by The American Legacy Foundation, an independent, public health organization created in 1999 as a result of the Master Settlement Agreement (MSA).

Q#24 "I HEARD THAT I SHOULD QUIT GRADUALLY OR IT COULD BE TOO MUCH OF A SHOCK FOR THE BABY. IS THAT TRUE?"

Spontaneously quitting or going "cold turkey" off nicotine is not too much for the baby to handle. Remember to put together a quit plan before you quit, as this will increase your chances of success. Maintain your own authority, which means doing what feels right for you.

Reminder: Finish off your quit plan and get ready for a quit date within the next two weeks. If you haven't written in that date yet do try and do so within the next 24 hours.

Q#25 "MY MOTHER SMOKED DURING ALL OF HER PREGNANCIES AND WE ALL TURNED OUT OKAY. WHY DO I NEED TO QUIT?"

Many of the risks of smoking during pregnancy were not as well researched or well known a generation ago, and your mom may not have been aware of many of the risks when she was raising her family. Today, we know there are many risks to the baby when a mother uses tobacco products.

Research into the risks associated with childhood exposure to second-hand smoke are ongoing. Although your parents' generation may have been unaware of the consequences of smoking around their children, we now have valuable information that can make a real impact on this next generation of children. By staying off tobacco products when you bring your baby home, you directly improve the chances that your baby will develop without complications potentially caused by tobacco products. The benefits of quitting and keeping your home smoke-free include the fact that your baby will have fewer colds, ear infections, and respiratory infections. Your baby will also be less likely to develop allergies.

If you quit smoking, you and the baby will enjoy many benefits. Imagine you have just met a person who promises:

- to give you better health,
- to give you thousands of dollars this year and every year, starting immediately, and
- to give you more time to enjoy your good health and money.

That person is you the day you quit using tobacco products.

The benefits of quitting.

1. Using tobacco during pregnancy causes low-birth-weight in one in five babies. Women who quit early in a pregnancy are less likely to have a low-birth-weight baby than those who continue to smoke. Low-birth-weight can cause complications and serious health issues for the baby.

2. Quitting decreases the risk of having an ectopic pregnancy and of the premature rupture of the membranes, separation of the placenta from the uterus and abnormal location of the placenta, which can result in serious complications.

3. You will breathe easier and you will have more energy.

Twenty minutes after quitting, your blood pressure and pulse will return to normal and the temperature in your extremities will normalize. Eight hours after quitting, the oxygen level in your blood will return to normal, which benefits both you and your baby. Within 48 hours your nerve endings will start to repair and your sense of smell and taste will have improved.

4. Your skin will look brighter.

5. Your breast milk will be free from the chemicals that lurk in tobacco products and this will result in the baby sleeping longer which will help with their development. In addition, your baby will be less likely to experience colic.

6. Quitting will help the baby's lungs grow strong.

7. You will lower the risk that your baby will be born prematurely. Premature birth can lead to potential problems with breastfeeding along with health issues.

8. Stopping smoking can reduce the risk of your child becoming obese later in life. Research shows that smoking leads to a subtle structural variation in the growing brain of the unborn baby that creates a preference for consuming fats. Studies suggest that maternal use of tobacco is a risk factor for obesity with maternal smoking defined as using more than one cigarette a day during the second trimester. Studies that reviewed brain scans of teens whose mothers used tobacco products while pregnant showed changes to the region of the brain that plays a role in processing emotions and storing memories.

9. You will have more money.

Exercise#10: *Calculating the money you will save.*
A big perk of quitting is that you will have more money to spend on your baby because you aren't spending on tobacco products. Consider this: The average cost of a pack of cigarettes in the United States is between $6.00 and $10.00. The average smoker smokes one pack a day or 20 cigarettes. Now add up your savings!

Cost per pack $ _____ x _____ packs per day = (A) $_____
(A)$ _____ x 7 days = (B) $ _____
(B)$ _____ x 39 weeks= (C) $ _____
(C) = Total savings during pregnancy =$ _____

(A sample cost savings for a pack a day over your pregnancy = $1,638.00)

Now consider that this is the amount you will save every nine months going forward.

Write down two to four items you either need or want to buy now that you have this extra money. (*Add this to your quit plan.*)
Revisit your list to remind yourself of what you can look forward to buying. Make sure you have some big-ticket items on it, because the amount of money you will be saving will be significant.
In addition to saving money, you will have more time to do other pleasant things or get some extra rest. It takes, on average, six minutes to smoke a cigarette and an additional three minutes before the smoke on your breath dissipates sufficiently to not

expose others to the effects of the second-hand smoke from the cigarette you just put out.

At a pack a day, that amounts to three hours every day devoted to the activity of smoking. If you stop smoking during the nine months of your pregnancy, you will have saved over one month's worth of time. If only you could trade those hours in for more sleep. Now that would be magical!

Risks of second-hand smoke.

There are two types of second-hand smoke: the smoke that is exhaled from a smoker's lungs and the smoke that comes off the end of a burning cigarette. Cigarettes and nicotine contain many harmful chemicals and they are present in both types of second-hand smoke. Every smoker needs to know that the chemicals added to cigarettes make them toxic. Protecting your baby starts with knowing what is in the products you buy. We demand it of our food products and we should demand nothing less from nicotine and tobacco products.

The definitive answer to the risk of using tobacco products.

"Decades of research have documented that smoking is a cause of cancer, heart disease, stroke, and chronic pulmonary disease, (29 USA Surgeon General's reports have documented the overwhelming and conclusive biologic, epidemiologic, behavioral and pharmacologic evidence that tobacco use is deadly." —US Department of Health and Human Services 2010.

"There is no safe level of exposure to tobacco smoke." —Regina Benjamin, MD, US Surgeon General.

Current research.

Two reports released in January 2013 emphasized the benefits of cessation for both sexes and noted the increased health risks for women who continue to use tobacco in comparison to the risks for men. When your mother was in her child-bearing years, many of the studies on tobacco use were focused on men as researchers did not have access to generations of long-term, regular female users of tobacco products. Fortunately, you can benefit from current studies in a multitude of disciplines. Current research, conducted on data collected between 1997 and 2004, provides the following findings:

- The women in this cohort represent the first generation of women in the United States to begin smoking early in life and to continue to do so for decades.
- The disease risks from cigarette smoking increased over most of the 20th century in the United States as successive generations of first male and then female smokers began smoking at progressively earlier ages.
- The relative risks of death from lung cancer, COPD, or any other cause among current smokers, as compared with those who had never smoked, increased according to the number of cigarettes smoked per day and the number of years they had been a smoker.

If you compare your own experience with smoking to your mother's, note not only when she started and how much she smoked, but also how tobacco products have changed over the years.

In a January 2013 editorial in *The New England Journal of Medicine*, Steven A. Schroeder, MD wrote "The hazard ratios for lung-cancer mortality were staggering; 17.8 for female smokers and 14.6 for male smokers. Also the risk of death for women who smoke is 50% higher than the estimates reported in the 1980's." He further commented:

> Beginning in 1995, smokers smoked fewer cigarettes per day. (Schroeder SA –*How clinicians can help smokers to quit*. JAMA 2012;308:1586-7). Thun et al. speculate that increasing death rates from chronic obstructive pulmonary disease among male smokers over the three time periods reflect design changes in cigarettes that allow deeper inhaling.

He concluded his editorial with a call for his profession to do more to encourage quit attempts and to pay more attention to the policies known to reduce the prevalence of smoking. He also offered a reminder that it is never too late to quit.

Author Jane E. Brody discussed changes in cigarettes in a blog entry at NYTimes.com on February 18, 2013. She noted:

> Furthermore, changes in how cigarettes are manufactured may have increased the dangers of smoking. The use of perforated filters, tobacco blends that are less irritating, and paper that is more porous made it easier to inhale smoke and encouraged deeper inhalation to achieve satisfying blood levels of nicotine.

You need to seriously place blame where it belongs in all of this—with the industry.

Thousands upon thousands of people throughout the world are working on how to help you stop smoking. Millions upon millions of dollars have been spent on the subject and will continue to be spent in an effort to create a tobacco-free generation and to help anyone who is ready to quit to get the help and support they need. For every person you may have encountered who couldn't give you what you needed or has been rude to you about this issue, there are thousands who have your back and dislike the industry every bit as much as you do.

Q#26 "WILL TRYING TO QUIT NOW THAT I AM PREGNANT PUT TOO MUCH PRESSURE ON ME AND POSSIBLY CAUSE DEPRESSION? I HAVE BEEN DEPRESSED IN THE PAST."

Between 10% and 25% of women develop depression at some time in their lives, and the risk is highest during a woman's childbearing years. Pregnancy is a known potential trigger for depression, possibly because of the hormonal and lifestyle changes that occur at this time. Studies have shown that between 7% and 13% of pregnant women will experience some level of depression. Further studies also have established that there is a cause and effect relationship between smoking and an increased risk of depression.

➤ PREGNANT WOMEN WITH DEPRESSION HAVE A HIGHER CHANCE OF EXPERIENCING POSTPARTUM DEPRESSION THAN THE GENERAL FEMALE POPULATION. IT IS ADVISABLE TO SEEK PROFESSIONAL MEDICAL ATTENTION EARLY ON IN YOUR PREGNANCY SO YOU CAN GET THE BEST PREVENTATIVE CARE POSSIBLE.

You should discuss any personal history of depression with your maternity healthcare team so they can offer you support and give you the most appropriate information. Depression can be a serious chronic illness. In addition to discussing your personal history with your medical team, you should also mention any current symptoms, including deep feelings of sadness, anxiety, irritability, fatigue, or thoughts of death or self-harming. Feelings of hopelessness or helplessness are very serious signs that you need someone to help you. Depression is very common in our stressful world but you can find help if you reach out to someone.

Most women will experience postpartum blues—or baby blues—in the early days after giving birth. This is a very normal occurrence and is not the same as postpartum depression. Postpartum blues are attributed to a lack of sleep, the expenditure of energy during labor, and changing hormones levels. When a mother begins breastfeeding, endorphins are released. These endorphins help to prevent the mother from experiencing further hormonal deprivation symptoms as her body adjusts to no longer being pregnant.

Planning ahead to make the first months at home run as smoothly as possible is always a good idea. It's even more important if you do not have family support or if you have a personal history of depression or anxiety. Doulas, if you are not familiar with the profession, offer support to a woman, and potentially her partner, during the pregnancy and at the birth. They can also be called upon to help with the care of the baby during the first weeks. Think Mary Poppins.

Proactive steps to make the first few months as stress-free as possible.

1. If possible, sleep when the baby sleeps. Try napping with the baby on your chest with your legs leaning up against a wall. This position rests your physical body and the closeness

between you and your baby will be comforting to you both. You could listen to music or just close your eyes as you lie in this position for a few minutes.

2. Get outside every day in the fresh air and walk around the block. Walking is a great stress-releaser.

3. Practice letting go. A very helpful practice is to close your eyes and imagine yourself sitting under a lovely tree in a quiet spot beside a stream. Let anything that comes along in your mind just slip off on a leaf and float off down the stream. This act of detaching, of letting go is outstandingly calming and is a form of meditation.

4. Focus on your breath. Remember to breathe slowly and deeply. Cup your hands over your ears and breathe deeply. Think of each breath as a wave lapping the sands of a beautiful beach.

5. Join new parent groups and make new friends who share a common interest in parenthood to build a support network.

6. Look forward to witnessing your baby's growth. Start a baby journal or write letters to your baby about your pregnancy. Write down your hopes and dreams for the future and the things you are looking forward to, such as reading your child their first book or planning their first birthday party. Imagine becoming a grandparent to your children's children.

All parents set out to do the best for their children but sometimes circumstances and events get in their way. Parenting is nothing if not humbling.

A very helpful resource for information on depression and pregnancy is *www.mothertobaby.org*.

Q#27 "WHEN IS IT OKAY TO RETURN TO ALCOHOL AFTER GIVING BIRTH? I ALSO WANT TO LIMIT THE BINGE DRINKING I WAS DOING BEFORE I BECAME PREGNANT."

A detailed conversation about alcohol overuse falls outside the scope of these pages, but if the amount or frequency of your consumption ever starts to become a problem, many of the ideas in this book may be useful in helping you curtail your drinking or even abstain. If your drinking patterns are disrupting your daily life, then it is strongly recommended that you reach out and find a community health agency or a skilled professional counselor who can help. Ideally, you should wait until you have finished breastfeeding before you reintroduce alcohol to your life.

Alcohol use in pregnancy and breastfeeding.

- If you drink alcohol during pregnancy, you put your baby at serious risk of health problems.
- Alcohol consumed by a mother can pass to the baby while nursing. Not drinking while breastfeeding is the safest strategy.
- If you drink alcohol and are breastfeeding, it is strongly recommended that you wait until the alcohol has cleared from your system before you nurse again to ensure the baby is not exposed. By using a prepared charting method that takes into consideration your weight and the number of drinks you have had or plan to have, you can estimate how long it takes for the alcohol to clear from your body.
- For a woman weighing 150 pounds, it takes four-and-a-half hours for two alcoholic drinks to clear sufficiently from her system not to affect a nursing baby.

- For a woman weighing 120 pounds, it takes two-and-a-half hours for one alcoholic drink to clear from her system.

Drinking beer to help establish breastfeeding is not a good idea for a number of reasons. During the first few days after the birth of the baby, many women experience "the baby blues." As alcohol is known to magnify presenting emotions, it is wise to hold off on any alcohol at this time and to find other ways to establish breastfeeding. Avoiding alcohol in the early days is also recommended for the benefit of the baby.

➤ PLANNING WHEN YOU WILL HAVE A DRINK AND HOW MANY YOU WILL HAVE IS THE KEY TO SAFE ALCOHOL CONSUMPTION. CHARTS ARE AVAILABLE ONLINE AT *WWW.MOTHERRISK.ORG.*

Controlling your alcohol consumption.

Here are some tips for setting limits on how you much and how often you drink:

- I will drink only on weekends, only every other day.
- I will never drink alone.
- I will never drink before five.
- I will set limits on the quantity I drink and stay within them.
- I will never drink and drive.
- I will have a glass of water before having a drink and a glass of water before having a second drink.
- Drink only with meals to curtail when and how much you drink.
- Ounce for ounce, wine has twice the calories of soda. Track your alcohol calories and incorporate those totals in a reasonable daily range for your health goals.
- Alcohol can interrupt sleep patterns. Don't drink too close to bedtime.

You cannot rely on alcohol to change how you feel. It cannot make you feel happy, give you confidence, take away stress, or reduce your anxiety. All it can do is magnify a presenting emotion. If you have had a very bad day, drinking alcohol could make you feel a whole lot worse or at best just make you feel numb. Alcohol cannot take your troubles away. Its effect on your mood has a great deal to with your state of mind when you have that first glass. Sitting at home and drinking after a terrible day versus going out with your friends to have a good time and drinking can result in two very different emotional outcomes. For this reason it is best not to use or rely on alcohol for coping with stress, anxiety, or depression.

If you start to use alcohol in an attempt to solve problems you may come to understand the true meaning of the phrase "one is too many and one thousand will never be enough." Drinking to relieve sorrows is a dangerous and treacherous path.

A question for you:

Would you drink and drive?

One reason individuals won't drink and drive is that they have already taken positive preventative steps by making it a rule to never drink and drive. Building a strong set of guidelines around drinking will reduce the risk of alcohol disrupting your life as you move forward.

Q#28 "I HAVE SWITCHED TO E-CIGARETTES. IS THAT A GOOD IDEA?"

Electronic cigarettes, or e-cigarettes, are battery-operated products that turn chemicals into a vapor that is inhaled by the user. They have been available since 2004, and were first introduced to North America in 2007. To date there are no reliable data to determine if they are safe for the general population or for pregnant women. There is also a lack of evidence about their effectiveness as a method of quitting smoking.

Information provided on the American Cancer Society website says:

> Information from the FDA suggests that e-cigarettes are not always safe. A 2009 analysis of 18 samples of cartridges from 2 leading e-cigarette brands found cancer-causing substances in half the samples.... Testing also found small amounts of nicotine in most of the cartridges labeled nicotine-free.

The drug nicotine brings many risks:

- Nicotine raises blood sugar.
- Nicotine causes high blood pressure and clogging of the arteries.
- Nicotine creates wrinkles.
- Nicotine increases a person's heart rate and blood pressure and can interfere with blood flow to the heart, increasing the risk of cardiovascular diseases.
- Nicotine affects the brain. It mimics naturally occurring brain chemicals, which can lead to addiction. A person who uses nicotine lives between the extremes of enough and a sense of depletion. The experience of withdrawal is the definition of addiction.
- Nicotine can have negative effects on muscles, including the muscles of your diaphragm which enable you to breathe properly. It can lead to abnormal twitching and paralysis.

- Nicotine can lead to a loss of brain functions and cause seizures.

There is serious concern that if youths use e-cigarettes, it may lead them to nicotine addiction and eventually to other nicotine products, such as cigarettes. It takes only the inhalation of one cigarette to program the brain for nicotine addiction and once addicted, does it really matter where the next hit of nicotine comes from as long as there is one? E-cigarettes do not contain tobacco and therefore they are not regulated by the same laws as cigarettes. They can be purchased online without the purchaser needing to disclose their age.

It is time for complete honesty, accountability, and disclosure.
1. The ingredients in e-cigarettes and tobacco products are not labeled.
2. "Tobacco products are the only legal consumer product that are lethal when used exactly as the manufacturer intends"—*www.quitsolutions.org.*
3. The ingestion of cigarettes can be lethal. All tobacco and nicotine products should be kept out of reach of children and pets.

Q#29 "I AM FACING PROBLEMS IN MY LIFE RIGHT NOW SO I CAN'T DEAL WITH QUITTING."

There is a significant difference between saying "No, not now," and "No, not ever." There is no need to push, not yet. Take slow and gentle breaths, leaving room for possibilities. If you cannot make a decision to stop smoking, try to cut down and set a date two weeks away to revisit the idea of quitting. As you read this book you will find general problem-solving strategies and constructive ways to handle stress. The mind and body work together and have a fascinating ability to relieve each other of the role of coping with stressful events if one or the other becomes overloaded. It is truly remarkable how the body and mind work in partnership. Just as the body uses distraction as a strategy, the mind can play tricks on itself to deflect a stressor in your life.

Here is a personal story that illustrates this point:

During a turbulent time in my life I started losing my keys on a regular basis. My many problems challenged my mental and emotional abilities and were pushing me into a chronic stress mode that had me losing sleep, biting my fingernails incessantly, and drinking too much. Instead of being flattened by the weight of financial ruin and the end of a traumatic relationship, my mind shifted to worrying about the whereabouts of the keys to my house and to my car and with that came a whole new set of problems: two trucks, locksmiths, and the related expenses. By creating these new problems my mind was distracted from the bigger, more menacing issues and what seemed like insurmountable problems. Each night as I lay in bed the bigger problems would come back to life. Life did get better but to this day I carry my keys on a large key ring and do whatever I can to avoid misplacing my keys.

We can think only one thought at a time and, if you are busy worrying about how you are going to get back into your house, other thoughts will fade to gray. We distract ourselves until we can find a way to solve our problems. Nail biting is a classic mind-body distraction.

Q#30 "HOW CAN FINDING SOMEONE TO HELP SUPPORT ME MAKE A DIFFERENCE?"

The word "support" is a tough one to define. Take some time and consider not only who is best suited to help you but also what support would look, sound like, and feel like to you. Answer the following question for a couple of individuals whom you know. You can do this here or in your journal or file.

If I felt supported in my effort to quit smoking this would be happening in my relationship with:

Name of individual.

What would support from this person sound like?

What would support from this person look like?

What would support from this person feel like?

Could you ask this person for this support?

How would you ask this person for specific support?

Support.

This is not about asking someone to take responsibility for you. You get to decide what you tell them and what you keep private.

Support can come in many forms. Getting some help with the shopping, errands, or cleaning your house could relieve the stress in your life and help a quit effort.

1. On your quit plan, list people with whom you would like to share your thoughts about smoking and quitting. Come back to it later with new names. Remember to look outside your immediate circle.

2. Plan to ask each of these people for their support.
3. Consider specific ways in which each of these people can best support you.
4. Ask friends to not smoke around you.
5. Ask your friends and partner to not smoke in the car and to not let anyone else smoke in the car.
6. Ask a friend or family member to go for a walk once a week.
7. Ask key people, or potentially difficult people, to be extra patient with you as get used to your new smoke-free lifestyle.
8. If you know when you might be tempted to smoke, find someone to keep you company. You can discuss quitting or not.
9. Ask someone to join you on a lunch break from work.
10. Ask someone to do something enjoyable at a break time that does not involve smoking.
11. Take the time to talk openly to the people in your life who might be affected by your decision to quit smoking or to cut down.
12. Ask for what you need in an assertive and positive way and point out what might not be helpful or could contribute to you starting smoking all over again. For example, "Please do not light up around me or ask me to carry your cigarettes in my purse when we go out."
13. Have the number of a smoking cessation support line available if you think it might help. Reach out for encouragement and support if you need it.

The gift of listening.

An empathetic listener is someone who hears what you have to say, appreciates your feelings, and understands what you are thinking.

It is estimated that our minds wander during 50% of our waking hours. A supportive listener can help to keep you centered and in the moment. We speak to ourselves at a rate of hundreds of words per minute and when we verbally express ourselves we are forced to slow down in order to be understood. This is a good thing. It gives us a chance to hear ourselves think and we come to better understand what is going on for us at any particular time.

It is reported that people search Google to inquire about how to speak four times as often as they search how to listen. Giving someone your time, really listening to them, to appreciate their thoughts and what they are experiencing, is a great way to show support when someone has asked for your help. People can be their own "best experts" who simply need an opportunity to be heard.

Exercise #11: Listening.

Ask another person to listen to you for five minutes and ask that they then share what they heard you say. You may want to use a script. Choose any of the questions below or create your own questions to get things started.

Possible questions:

1. What do you enjoy about smoking?
2. What are the benefits of smoking?
3. Give five reasons why you smoke.
4. Give five reasons why you wish you didn't smoke.
5. Will you quit eventually?
6. What does success look like to you?

Now change roles and become the listener. Offer to listen to someone with a personal problem or a decision to make. Here are the guidelines:

1. Agree that what you say or hear is confidential.
2. Share your personal experience only if asked. Don't give advice unless asked.
3. Treat the person with respect and kindness, and show compassion. Try and see and feel the situation from their point of view. "Wear their shoes."
4. Let the other person speak without interruption and only interrupt if you need clarification of a point.

Q#31 "HOW CAN I RESPOND TO CRITICISM THAT I HAVE NOT BEEN ABLE TO QUIT?"

If you are in a heated discussion and get to the point where you wish to end the discussion, you can do so at any time by calmly saying, "I am not finding this conversation to be helpful."

If the other person becomes aggressive, end the conversation by saying, "This conversation is over." With the message delivered, you can then leave without getting sucked into the other person's negativity and you will avoid escalating the situation.

"Even when a situation seems so personal, even if others insult you directly, it has nothing to do with you. What they say, what they do, and the opinions they give are according to the agreements they have in their own minds. When you truly understand this, and refuse to take things personally, you can hardly be hurt by the careless comments or actions of others." —Don Miguel Ruiz

Constructive criticism has its place. If you have asked for someone's opinion, it is best to be prepared to hear what that person has to say. If their remarks are not useful, you can either choose to end the conversation or ask them to explain why they felt the need to express their remarks. Asking someone to tell you why they said something can help to keep the conversation open and more honest.

You may have had direct experience of hearing a former smoker's frustration with current smokers. They cannot understand why anyone would continue to smoke given all that is known about the health risks.

People who do not smoke are able to objectively look at the risks of smoking and accept this information. It validates their beliefs. It is unimaginable that they would ever light up and they may pat themselves on the back for being so responsible. For people who don't smoke, there is only one clear and undeniable choice: if you smoke, quit.

For a person who smokes, the situation is very different. Faced with the news bulletins about the health risks, the person who smokes has a dilemma. If they have been unable to quit and have failed at numerous quit attempts, they may have decided that they will never be able to quit. With this in mind, they have to reject the idea that ongoing smoking is harmful and have to buy into the belief system that they will beat the odds. If you think about it, what other choice can a person who smokes make and remain positive about their future?

This is what people who don't smoke find so difficult. They are asking people who don't believe they can quit—or at least have not found success yet—to buy into a belief system that is extremely limiting when there is another belief system that offers someone who smokes a way out: there is a chance of beating the odds that smoking will cause death.

It isn't even necessary for the person who smokes to reject

both outcomes or to deny the odds. They leave their options open and see a way out, which is hardly surprising when you consider the topic is so dire.

People are not equally adversely affected by the use of tobacco products because of genetics, other lifestyle choices, circumstances, and age. All these factors affect the development of the diseases and ailments linked to the use of tobacco products.

Q#32 "WHAT ARE THE BEST REASONS FOR QUITTING?"

Quitting for financial reasons is a great reason because you are spared the health lectures and it is 100% guaranteed that you will save money when you stop. "I quit because it became too expensive." End of conversation, end of story.

Money is one of the top answers given by former smokers when asked why they quit.

Here are the reasons people often give for deciding to quit:

1. A current health problem.
2. A change of lifestyle.
3. A new partner or roommate.
4. Advised to quit by healthcare provider.
5. Pressured to quit by coworkers.
6. Pressured to quit by family.
7. Peer pressure.
8. Disgusted by the smell.
9. Tired of the hassle.
10. Lack of enjoyment.
11. Consideration of future health.
12. Pregnancy or family planning.

13. Concern about the health of a friend or family member.
14. Smoking-related illness of a friend or family.

It is interesting to note that 15.40% of women and 55% of men said the fear of premature aging made them quit, with 25% of women and 10% of men wanting to stop to increase their chances of having a baby. 25% of men report quitting after being diagnosed with some form of erectile dysfunction. Nicotine restricts blood flow in the body which can impact sexual and reproductive function and capacity.

Fewer than one in three successful quitters say a concern for their future health was the reason they quit, and yet it is interesting that this is where most non-smokers focus in their discussions with people who they wish would stop smoking.

Visit your quit plan and list your personal reasons for wanting to quit.

Q#33 "HOW CAN I GET OTHER PEOPLE WHO WILL BE AROUND THE BABY TO UNDERSTAND THE RISKS OF SECOND-HAND AND THIRD-HAND SMOKE?"

You need to ask for what you want to happen. And you need to be direct about it.

As the child's mother, you have the right to ask for changes that will give your baby the best possible chances, and that includes limiting smoking in your environment. Using positive "I"-based statements when communicating with your family and friends will help produce good results. Of course, the opposite is true if your requests become passive or aggressive.

What is the difference between being assertive, being passive, and being aggressive? An assertive request starts with the phrase "I need your help," or "I need you to know," followed by a brief explanation of your desire to have a healthy environment for you and the baby. You may need to tactfully educate your family and friends about the chemicals in tobacco products and the consequences of exposure to smoking. Passive communication is suffering in silence and not speaking up for what you want to happen. Aggressive communication is argumentatively demanding that everyone around you quit smoking immediately. Neither passive language nor aggressive language will likely get you the results you want.

Ask for what you need. For example, if your parents or parents-in-law smoke, you could start the conversation by saying "I need your help in providing a smoke-free home, car, and living space. You may not know that some of the chemicals in cigarettes and in second-hand smoke are harmful to all of us. Did you know that it takes weeks to clear a room of residual chemicals from smoking? I would like to discuss how we can work this out together to create a healthy environment so the baby and I can visit your home and the child can have a close relationship with their grandparents."

The risks of second-hand smoke.

1. There are three components of second-hand smoke: the smoke coming off the tip of a lit cigarette, the air exhaled by a person who is smoking, and the chemicals that escape through the cigarette wrapper of a lit cigarette.
2. There are thousands of chemical compounds in second-hand smoke. Of these, 200 are poisons and more than 69 cause cancer.

3. Studies show that children with a parent who smokes around them get sick more often. Their lungs grow less than those of children who are not exposed to second-hand smoke, and they get bronchitis and pneumonia more frequently, along with being at greater risk for meningitis, ear infections and dental cavities.

4. Worldwide, more than 600,000 non-smokers die each year from exposure to second-hand smoke.

5. In a study of babies with parents who smoked on average 76 cigarettes a week, scientists detected cancer-causing chemicals associated with tobacco smoke in the urine of 50% of those babies.

6. Infants of non-smoking parents have the lowest risk of Sudden Infant Death Syndrome (SIDS). The risk of SIDS is lower for infants whose mothers stopped smoking while pregnant.

Third-hand smoke.

Third-hand smoke is the residual tobacco smoke that lands on items and stays there after a cigarette has been put out. Tar and nicotine particles linger on surfaces, including clothing, hair, furniture, car upholstery, and pet fur. Over time, these particles can release 200 poisonous gases and they have been linked to cancer.

For three minutes after smoking a cigarette, residuals on a person's breath and clothing can contaminate a space that they enter.

It can then take up to two weeks for a previously safe, closed interior space to become safe again after having been contaminated with tobacco smoke. Hazardous carcinogens result when the nicotine in tobacco smoke reacts with nitrous acid (a common component of indoor air). These carcinogens are created over time—days and weeks—and can be inhaled, absorbed, or ingested.

Q#34 "I HAVE NO SELF-CONTROL AND DON'T BELIEVE I CAN DO THIS LONG-TERM."

Chrissy's own concerns may help you with this problem. Chrissy has a really tough job and she relies on her smoke-breaks to make it through the day. She hasn't given up on the idea of quitting but doesn't think she has what it takes. She believes she has no self-control. Her information is paralyzing and incorrect. In fact, she must have self-control as she deals with nicotine's demands approximately every 30 to 45 minutes.

If she really had no self-control, she would stop whatever she was doing—pleasurable or not—to deal with this relentless and demanding drug every 30 to 45 minutes. But she does not stop what she's doing. Instead, she gets on with her day and smokes when she can conveniently do so, which is at smoke-break, lunch, and after work. She is in charge and exercises self-control whenever she denies or delays the drug's call.

If she really did not have any self-control, then every 30 minutes, during work, while sleeping, while making love, in the middle of great movie, she would go outside, whether the weather was fair or foul and regardless of what anyone around her thought, and she would smoke. We use self-control all day long in every aspect of our lives. It is part of our human survival mechanism. It keeps us safe as well as socially acceptable.

Addictive drugs like tobacco products may call your name, but you can and do deny them and you do it from a place of self-control.

Human beings are hardwired with self-control. If you did not have self-control, the drug would have the power to drag you out on command. Yes, this is an addictive drug but you have free will and your beliefs, which you do have control over, play a significant role in your ongoing usage. It just takes time to slow down and work out which beliefs are limiting you and then challenge them head on.

The "big factors."

> THE DRUG NICOTINE FOOLS THE PERSON INTO THINKING THAT THE NEXT CIGARETTE BRINGS RELAXATION WHEN, IN FACT, THE NEXT CIGARETTE BRINGS RELIEF FROM THE FEELING OF NICOTINE DEPLETION. IT IS A VICIOUS CIRCLE.

Take extra care not to turn the "big factors" into excuses for not deciding to quit or, if you have quit, making them your reasons for slipping back.

"I suffer from low self-esteem. That is why I can't quit." Look for practical solutions to the problems you face and not over-whelming ideas that you may have no way of proving let alone solving. Stick to solid strategies worth trying.

"Nicotine has altered my brain chemistry and it will take months or years to undo the damage." You can take this day by day and step by step. Let each day define itself. Remind yourself that millions upon millions of people have achieved this. You can be one of them.

"This is addiction." If you find yourself feeling helpless and the situation seems hopeless, consider changing the dynamics. Get hold of the anger you feel in response to the influence this ugly force has had over your life and fight back with everything you have. Nicotine will try all kinds of tricks to keep you hooked, even B.R.A.T. tactics (Boundary Resistant Addiction Tantrum). This is when you need to stand your ground. Use your creativity to mount a campaign to win back your freedom. Remember to ensure that your ideas work in your favor and do not create any additional stress for you or your baby.

Join the Campaign for Tobacco-Free Kids and participate in their activities to push back tobacco. Be proactive in the fight for a tobacco-free generation.

Start a collection of quotes or inspirational sayings that resonate with your thoughts and feelings. Here are some that you may find helpful to carry with you:

"There are no neurotics or geniuses or failures or fools. There are only neurotic moments, flashes of brilliance, failed opportunities and stupid mistakes. But these moments, pleasant or unpleasant can never fix us into rigid immutable characters. We cannot help but change."
—David Reynolds

"Most people fail in the art of living, not because they are inherently bad or so without will that they cannot lead a better life: They fail because they do not wake up and see when they stand in the fork in the road and have to decide."
—Erika Fromm

"Show me a day when the world wasn't new."
—Sister Barbara Hance

"When you get to the end of your rope tie a knot in it, and hang on."
—President Thomas Jefferson

Q#35 "WHAT CAN I DO OR SAY THAT WILL HELP MY DAD? HE WANTS TO QUIT BUT THE TOPIC MAKES HIM UNCOMFORTABLE."

Let your dad know you understand and appreciate how he feels. Here are some suggestions on how to support him:

- Ask if he would like your help. It's important to check that he wants your advice before offering it. Children can have a particularly difficult time stepping into their parents' affairs. Go slowly. For example, you could open up the conversation by saying, "I am here for you if you want to talk about quitting. I would be happy to help you. If there is something I can do to help please let me know. I am happy to share what worked for me and what strategies I used."

- Encourage him to discuss why quitting is personally relevant at this time. Remind yourself that anyone can have the best of reasons in mind and still not change.

- Listen to what he is saying about quitting, and about his thoughts and feelings. Ask him open-ended questions. For example, you could ask him, "What have you tried before that worked?"

- Remind him that many other people have been in this position and you understand that millions eventually found a way to quit. Mention that it often took them several attempts.

- Share things that were helpful to you and that could also be appropriate for him.

- Respect that he may find ways to quit that are very different from those you tried.

Q#36 "MY MOM HAS NEVER SMOKED AND HAS NO PATIENCE FOR ANYONE WHO DOES. WHAT CAN I SAY THAT WILL HELP HER TO UNDERSTAND WHAT I AM GOING THROUGH?"

People who have never used tobacco products do not have the benefit of experience. You may need to help them to understand the challenges of quitting. It may be very helpful to share with your mother the facts about quitting from these pages that you found the most interesting.

Understanding drug addiction-dependency.

Nicotine is the addictive ingredient in cigarettes that plays with a person's mind. It tricks people into thinking that they need to keep using it. People who use tobacco products may believe they need a cigarette (nicotine) to handle the following situations:

- To concentrate.
- To deal with stressful, painful, or unpleasant situations.
- To relax.
- To cope with boredom.
- To stay alert.
- To avoid withdrawal symptoms.
- To avoid uncomfortable situations or feelings.
- To go to sleep or to wake up.
- To reduce anxiety in social situations.

The process of quitting.

Share the following tips with anyone who wants to help:

- Supporting a pregnant woman in her quit attempt means understanding her needs, thoughts, and feelings as she goes through the physical, emotional, and social stages of quitting.

- Ask how you can best help. Resist offering advice before it is asked for.
- Listen to her. Aim to understand what she is feeling and thinking.
- Encourage her by joining her in exercise and other healthy lifestyle activities.
- Tell her in many ways that she is strong enough to do this and that you believe she will succeed.
- Offer to talk about quitting and what she has been reading or has learned about quitting. Ask her to tell you what is working and the details of her plan. Take an interest in her quitting if your interest is well received.
- Increase her happiness factor.
- Never use the expression "It is hard to quit." This will not help.
- Never put things in terms of ultimatums.
- Drop the blame or shame talk, or any language that might be taken as producing guilt.
- Do not compare her to other people.
- Do not let anyone else smoke around her or the baby. Be their first line of defense.
- Do not offer her a cigarette.
- If she slips, remember that this is her process and treat her with loving kindness.
- Hold off with the "lectures."

Q# 37 "MY FIVE-YEAR-OLD DAUGHTER SAID SHE THINKS SMOKING IS STUPID. DOES THIS MEAN SHE WON'T SMOKE LATER AS A TEENAGER?"

However great a job parents and educators have done at raising young children's awareness of the dangers of tobacco use, we live in a world that continues to send mixed messages to our children about the use of tobacco products.

- "The use of tobacco products is risky."
- "Kids experiment and are rebellious against authority."
- "Quitting smoking is hard to do."
- "There are products that as an adult you can use to help you quit."
- "For every cigarette there is a Nicorette." (But only when you reach adulthood as they are not recommended for youth.)

Children start using tobacco products for a variety of reasons, including the fact that North American culture reinforces the pursuit of external gratification, quick fixes, and a reliance on a never-ending stream of experts along with "the next best things" that product marketers can send our way. Children are attracted to the activities and practices of their favorite role models who include movie stars and the faces beaming out from the glossy pages of magazines. But most damaging is the exploitation of a child's idea of their own invincibility, one of our finest human capacities, by the powerful industry that manufactures and markets nicotine.

Every day, more than 3,800 persons younger than 18 years of age smoke their first cigarette in the United States. Every day, about 1,000 persons younger than 18 years of age begin smoking daily in the United States.

Young adults, teens, and children who start experimenting with smoking may not know that over half of all smokers wish they could find a way to get tobacco products out of their lives. Some research puts the want-to-quit rate as high as 95%.

Young people also may not know that each year more than half of people who smoke try to quit but at any one time only 5% to 10% of people who smoke will manage to sustain their last quit attempt.

Do kids who start smoking understand what they are getting into when they light up to fit in with their peers?

Despite their relatively short smoking histories, many adolescents who smoke are nicotine dependent, and such dependence can lead to daily smoking. To examine the extent to which high school students had tried to quit smoking cigarettes, CDC analyzed data from the 2007 Youth Risk Behavior Survey (YRBS), a nationally representative survey of students in grades 9 to 12 in the United States. The report found that 60.9% of students who ever smoked cigarettes daily tried to quit smoking cigarettes, and 12.2% were successful. More students in 9th grade (22.9%) than in 10th grade (10.7%) 11th grade (8.8%) and 12th grade (10.0%) tried to quit smoking cigarettes and were successful.

Do kids know the true extent of the dangers conclusively linked to use of tobacco products or that tobacco prevention funding has been cut back in recent years in both the United States and Canada?

When the Tobacco Master Settlement Agreement was signed in 1998, a significant portion of the hundreds of billion dollars was to be used by the individual states over 25 years to attack the public health problems created by tobacco use. Reports from 2012 show individual states have cut their funding for tobacco prevention and cessation programs to levels not seen since the first settlement funds were paid out.

The states this year (Fiscal Year 2012) will collect $25.6 billion in revenue from the tobacco settlement and tobacco taxes, but will spend only 1.8 percent of it—$456.7 million—on programs to prevent kids from smoking and help smokers quit. This means the states are spending less than two cents of every dollar in tobacco revenue to fight tobacco use. Tobacco companies spend nearly $23 to market tobacco products for every $1.00 the states spend to fight tobacco use. According to the latest data from the Federal Trade Commission, tobacco companies spend $10.5 billion a year on marketing. (Campaign for Tobacco-Free Kids—A broken promise to our children.)

How children view the use of tobacco products.

98% of all children between the ages of 7 and 14 with parents who use tobacco products wish their parents would stop.

94% of children think smoking is either stupid or dangerous.

93% of children say they don't want their own children smoking when they grow up.

91% of children say they will never try a cigarette.

88% of children wish nobody in the world smoked.

73% of children with a parent who smokes worry about the risk of their parent dying.

33% of children with parents who smoke admit they have hidden their parents' cigarettes in an attempt to help them quit.

Many of these same children will be weaned off their dislike of tobacco products by the time they reach their youth and will become the industry's new lifelong clients.

Every day, more than 1,200 people in the United States die from a tobacco-generated disease. For each of those deaths, each and every day at least two youth or young adults become regular users of tobacco products. Tobacco products continue to be the chief preventable cause of disease, disability, and premature death in the United States.

➤ 22.4% OF WOMEN OF REPRODUCTIVE AGE IN AMERICA CURRENTLY SMOKE.

Q#38 "WHAT ROLE DO HORMONES PLAY IN QUITTING?"

Certain physiological factors in pregnancy, including the fluctuation in hormones, can explain a new reaction to particular scents and tastes, including tobacco products and coffee.

The role of fluctuating hormones, however, cannot adequately explain how many women end long-standing addictions to tobacco or a number of other substances when they learn they are pregnant. For these women, it is not hormonal changes but rather a realization that they must make a decision about their lifestyle choices that makes them act, and the powers of the imagination, beliefs, and a leap of faith come into play.

Women return to tobacco products after weeks or months of being free because they have not broken away from their attachment to these products. By taking the time now to fully question your relationship with tobacco and nicotine, you can take the required steps to create a belief system that considers returning to using tobacco products after the arrival of the baby as truly unimaginable.

We know that, over time, smoking will alter a person's brain cells and that it can take years after quitting for the brain to return to normal. We also know that there have been millions upon millions of people who have quit smoking and, once free of the drug, have gone on to live smoke-free and craving-free. For these successful quitters, something had to radically change about how they came at smoking. They had to change the way they thought about tobacco products. If you ask people who have quit how they did it, you will be surprised by the consistency in their answers.

Q#39 "I AM IN MY THIRD TRIMESTER AND SMOKING. MY PARTNER IS MAD AT ME AND I CAN'T HANDLE THIS CONFLICT. HELP!"

Look behind anger and you will find fear. Look behind fear and you will find what someone holds dear or loves. We defend or fight for something we feel is being threatened or think we are at risk of losing.

Ask yourself: What is he trying to defend? What is he trying to protect and what does he fear is at risk?

Approach conflict with an intense interest in getting to what the other person needs or wants to see happen and then take the time to find a way to help them to understand what you need. This is an opportunity to extend loving kindness.

When reading about specific tactics used by the tobacco industry earlier in this book, you may have felt annoyance or outright rage. Anger may have given you a charge of energy, a new surge of motivation to do something proactive in retaliation. Your anger may have contributed to a new resolve to stop buying tobacco products and to encourage others to do the same. Anger is a very energizing emotion that can drive us to make changes in our world. It is something to be embraced, not shut off. Anger—along with fear and all other emotions—is an emotion to be acknowledged and experienced. Our emotions play a large role in keeping us safe by giving us a "heads-up."

Have you ever had someone say to you, "Oh, please don't be angry. Please don't feel that way." Feelings are either denied or expressed but they cannot be directly controlled. We can choose to do things that will have an indirect effect on how we feel or how someone else feels. We cannot turn our colorful emotional worlds on and off on command and we certainly cannot directly determine how someone else will feel or act.

However, we have control over what we choose to do in any given situation. We get to decide what our next step and direction will be. Knowing that we have this power over our own behavior allows us the freedom to fully experience our feelings. Personal power is rooted in knowing our limits, knowing our boundaries, and knowing where to draw the line on our own behavior and on what we will or will not put up with from others.

How you deal with conflict.

In a good relationship, individuals enjoy each other's company, and all goes along smoothly until—inevitably—conflict arises. In conflict, one of two things will likely happen. Both parties will fight fairly, working through the presenting issue with mutual regard, respect, and understanding. Or one or both of the individuals will cross boundaries and the situation will be thrown off the rails. A stream of sarcastic comments, or belittling or personal remarks will escalate the conflict and little or nothing will be resolved.

In conflict between adults, fighting fair means there are rules, such as no personal insults and no aggression.

If your partner or someone you know crosses the line, recognize that you need to use your own power to end the discussion. Tell the person directly and calmly that the conversation is over, at least for now, and that they will need to "fight fair" or you will not continue. If your partner acts like this around you, it may be tempting to shrug it off with a list of excuses—for example, they were tired or having a bad day. There are no excuses for name calling, verbal abuse, accusations, or personal insults. Ever.

Asking for help.

If you think quitting smoking or making other lifestyle changes could cause serious conflict in a relationship and you do not think you will be able to handle it alone, you must get someone to help you. Put smoking to the side and take care of yourself. Seek help in addressing any situation or relationship in which you feel undermined or threatened. You do not need to do it alone. Well-trained people are available to help. They may have been in a similar situation to the one you now face and will be able to understand what you are going through and to offer valuable help. Tell your primary caregiver, your physician or midwife, and ask for their help in finding you the support you need.

Note: Interpersonal partner violence may begin or intensify during pregnancy. It is estimated that 40% of first incidents of interpersonal partner violence occur when the women is pregnant.

Q#40 "MY PARTNER WANTS TO QUIT. WHAT CAN I DO TO HELP?"
"Of the many cues that influence behavior, at any point in time, none is more common than the actions of others." —Albert Bandura

A new mother who is quitting has been proven to be the strongest influence on a new father being able to quit as well.

Keep sharing what you have discovered about quitting in an objective manner without adding pressure. A little of the right information at the right time can work wonders. Offer concrete information and give him the facts. Frequently, dads-to-be miss out on receiving valuable information about the risks associated with smoking around their pregnant partners. It is a great idea to share what you know with him and to invite him to attend healthcare appointments with you so he can meet the individuals whom you have found to be helpful.

Studies show that only 33% of new fathers are aware that the use of tobacco products contributes to SIDS, 24% understand that it contributes to ear infections, 65% know it is related to babies' developing asthma, bronchitis, and pneumonia, and 75% know it contributes to coughing/sore throats in babies.

Let your partner know that you are thrilled to be tobacco-free and that you are there for him any time to talk about quitting. Ask if he would like to look through *Baby & Me—Tobacco Free* and mark some pages that he might find interesting. Let him know that the risk of relapse is heightened by the number of individuals who smoke in a person's social network and if the person's partner continues to smoke. Together, you can do this. It is absolutely possible to quit smoking. This is where you begin.

FINAL COMMENT

When you wake up each day, take a moment and feel the ease of your breathing in your body. Acknowledge the strength of your resolve and how great it is that you ended this problem for yourself and made a real difference in the lives of the people you share your life with.

In order to repel the advances of the tobacco industry and save an estimated 1 billion lives this century, it will take a social cure, and the involvement of individuals, parents, educators, public health agencies, governments, and the movers and shakers of culture to halt the tobacco epidemic we face.

"Governments must make it their top priority to stop the tobacco industry's shameless manipulation of young people and women, in particular, to recruit the next generation.... " Dr. Margaret Chan, WHO Director-General May 31st. 2013 World No Tobacco Day. Support the banning of tobacco advertising, promotion and sponsorship.

PART THREE: YOUR QUIT PLAN

"To laugh often and much, to win the respect of intelligent people and the affection of children, to earn the appreciation of honest critics and endure the betrayal of false friends, to appreciate beauty, to find the best in others, to leave the world a bit better, whether by a healthy child, a garden patch. . . . to know even one life has breathed easier because you have lived. This is to have succeeded."—Ralph Waldo Emerson

Before your quit date arrives, make sure you have completed the preparation steps so that you have a solid foundation to support your efforts and help you reach your goal.

As you break free from tobacco you will reap noticeable benefits. You will feel better, breathe better, sleep better, cope better with stress, and feel remarkably more confident about your future. By following the suggestions outlined in this book you can take charge of your life and seize the opportunity to tell the people behind the tobacco industry that they do not deserve your money or your time. You might even want to join the authors of this book in suggesting that anyone working in the industry consider alternative employment while they still have time.

MAKING A DECISION TO QUIT

In the notebook or journal in which you created your quit plan, take notes on what works and the steps you took to quit.

1. Review pages 46–50.
2. Write a personal statement about your commitment to quitting.
3. Write the date you have chosen to quit. Set the date within the next two weeks, allowing sufficient time for you to be well prepared. Review page 51.
4. Review the benefits of quitting on page 93.
5. Write out the major benefits of quitting.
6. Write out your reasons for quitting.
7. Identify people who can help you in your quit effort. They will be your champions, encouraging you to stay smoke-free, even on a tough day. Tell your family and friends that you have chosen to quit smoking and ask for their support. List your supporters.
8. Identify the people whom you need to talk to about second-hand smoke. In an assertive, clear, firm, and kind voice, practice what you might say to them if you are feeling unsure of yourself. Practice the example scripts on page 115.

Others ways of getting support.
- Ask others not to smoke around you.
- Tell your doctor or healthcare provider you are quitting and ask if they can recommend resources or extra services you can access if you think that will help.
- Consider contacting a State Quitline to receive their support. Remember to tell them you are pregnant.

- Ask your supporters to remind you how well you are doing by not smoking.

PREPARING TO QUIT

1. Make your home and car smoke-free. There is no safe exposure level when it comes to second-hand smoke. You and your baby must be protected. Arrange to have your car and home tobacco-free and cleaned between 5 and 10 days before your quit date. Once your car and home are smoke-free, limit smoking to outside the car and house.

2. Prepare for the first day of quitting by throwing out all lighters, cigarettes, and ashtrays.

3. Take some quiet time and write out your plans for the next few days. Write out a plan with as much detail as feels comfortable.
   - *Example*: "At work I will spend my breaks taking a real break not a smoke-break. I will use this time to call a friend, eat a meal, and get some fresh air. When I get home from work I will have a shower. I will then plan a favorite meal and go for a walk around the block with my partner. In the evening I will plan to watch a favorite show and get a good night's sleep. If I have trouble falling asleep I am going to focus on my breathing. If I find myself having trouble with any urges to use tobacco I am going to call my sister or remember to sit down and find my breath."
   - *Example*: "On day one I have the day off from work so I am going to clean my kitchen. In the afternoon I am going to take a long bath and meet my friend and

do some shopping for new maternity clothes. In the evening I am going out to dinner and a movie with my partner and a couple of friends. I am also going to book a massage for tomorrow."

Stressors and triggers.

1. Remind yourself that non-smokers also experience stress. They find ways to handle that stress and you will too. In a journal, write down the tips or strategies that you want to remember to use when you encounter stress. Mark a page with the word STRESS across the top and plan to track when you become stressed or when you felt your self-control slipping away. When the stress episode has passed, note what you did to reduce your stress levels.
2. Review pages 58–64 on handling stress.
3. Plan ahead to avoid falling back into smoking. Write down your previous triggers, being around other people who are smoking, particular times of the day, for example.
4. Review the top three tips for dealing with stress on page 62.
5. Take deep, even breaths.
6. Get plenty of rest.
7. Take walks in the fresh air regularly.

Withdrawal.

Write down in detail how you will manage withdrawal symptoms if they arise.

Review pages pages 82–87.

Remember to use the Five "D's" on page 48.

Quit Day: Embrace the fact that you are now a non-smoker.
Tell yourself that you are ready. Remind yourself that you have put a good deal of time into preparing for this quit attempt and your efforts will pay off. Tell yourself that this time things will be different. Write in your journal each day about your experiences as you move further and further away from tobacco products.

Living a tobacco-free life.
1. Congratulate yourself often. You have successfully quit smoking and are excited to bring your healthy baby home to a smoke-free environment.
2. Never take even a puff of another cigarette or tobacco or nicotine product.
3. Don't buy cigarettes for others.
4. Think of yourself as a non-smoker.
5. Do not make deals with the voices in your head that may tempt you to start again.
6. Revisit page 95 to calculate how much money you are saving. Look at these figures often.
7. If you do slip, pick yourself up, brush yourself off, and remember that a slip is not a disaster if you get right back on the path to quitting.
8. Live the success. When you walk past someone smoking, enjoy the sense of relief you feel now that this problem is out of your life for good.

YOU have accomplished breaking free from the nicotine cycle and can rightfully cheer "I am, baby and me, tobacco free." Congratulations!

PART FOUR: RESOURCES

RECOMMENDED READING

The Hero Within by Carol S. Pearson, Harper One, New York, N.Y., 1998.

The Four Agreements—A Practical Guide to Personal Freedom by Don Miguel Ruiz, Amber-Allen Publishing San Rafael, California USA, 1997

The Cigarette Century—The Rise, Fall and Deadly Persistence of the product that defined America by Allan Brandt Basic Books New York 2007

Full Catastrophe Living by Jon Kabat-Zinn, Ph.D The Program of the Stress Reduction Clinic at the University of Massachusetts Medical Center. Dell Publishing 1990

Willpower – Rediscovering The Greatest Human Strength by Roy F. Baumeister and John Tierney The Penguin Press New York 2011

The Birth Partner by Penny Simkin,P.T. The Harvard Common Press, Boston, Massachusetts, 2008

A Handbook for Constructive Living by David K. Reynolds, PH.D. William Morrow and Company, Inc. New York 1995

CONTACTS
Baby&Me—Tobacco Free
http://www.babyandmetobaccofree.org
www.facebook.com/BabyandMeTF
Twitter: babyandmehealth

The Center for Disease Control (CDC) http://www.cdc.gov/
http://www.cdc.gov/tobacco/osh/organization/
The World Health Organization (WHO)
http://www.who.int/cancer/prevention/en/

UNITED STATES
National Quit Lines smokefree.gov 1-800-Quit-Now
http://www.smokefree.gov

CANADA
http://www.smokershelpline.ca/ 1-877-513-5333
Truth about the tobacco industry. http://www.thetruth.com
Spontaneous quitting. www.whyquit.com

Alcohol or any other exposure during pregnancy or breastfeeding: CTIS Pregnancy Health Information Line at 800-532-3749 or via instant message counseling at CTISPregnancy.org or by calling information specialists (OTIS) at 866-626-6847.

Prenatal care:
http://www.marchofdimes.com/pregnancy/prenatalcare.html

Free support on pregnancy and baby care
http://www.text4baby.com

Second hand smoke: http://www.aware.on.ca/starss

Labor support doulas: http://www.dona.org/

The author: http://www.youcanstopsmokingnow.com

The publisher: http://graftonandscratch.com
Twitter: gspublisher

SHAPING UP FOR A HEALTHY PREGNANCY

Bonnie Berk, MS, RN, HNB-BC, E-RYT, RPYT, is a board-certified holistic nurse. She is a pioneer in using yoga as a complementary therapy for people with cancer and chronic diseases. In 1980 she founded the Motherwell Maternity Fitness Program. She also developed the Motherwell Yoga DVD and Baby's Breath two-CD set for pregnant women planning for a healthy pregnancy and positive childbirth experience.

Exercise is a proven stress reliever. Taking walks on most days of the week will elevate your mood and prepare your body for the changes that occur in pregnancy. If you are already exercising, then it is recommended you walk or engage in aerobic exercise for 30 to 45 minutes a day at a pace that lets you talk in a comfortable, natural manner. However, if you are new to exercise, take it slowly. Start to walk for 10 to 15 minutes twice a day and build up slowly. Stretch after walking, paying especial attention to your leg muscles, the calves, quadriceps, and hamstrings. Low backstretches are also helpful in preventing back discomfort. You may also continue attending fitness classes, but try to exercise at a moderate intensity once you become pregnant. If you are not currently engaged in any strength or flexibility program, the following exercises will help you become strong, stretched, and centered. If you are already taking an exercise class or doing strengthening and flexibility exercises, add these to your routine.

Belly breathing

Sit, stand, or lie on your back in a comfortable position. Keep a neutral spine and take a deep breath, expanding the belly. During exhalation, pull the belly button toward the spine. Repeat 12 times, rest, and repeat another 12 times. Try to practice this exercise throughout the day when you are sitting in traffic or waiting in line at the bank or the grocery store.

Rounded cat stretch

On your knees and hands, assume a tabletop position. Check with your hands to make sure your back is straight. Take a breath. As you exhale, tighten your abdominal muscles, perform a posterior pelvic tilt, tuck the chin in, and round your back. During inhalation, make a "hollow cat back" while keeping the abdomen firm. Continue this exercise for 12 breath cycles and then rest with buttocks on heels and arms stretched out above the crown of the head (child's pose). Repeat for another 12 breath cycles.

Kegel exercises

Core strength includes the pelvic floor. In addition to strengthening the torso, practicing Kegel exercises will help you prevent leakage of urine during and after pregnancy and help restore muscle tone after delivery. Take a deep breath. On the exhale, squeeze the muscles around the vaginal opening and hold.

(When contracting these muscles, imagine pulling the vaginal opening up toward the inside of the navel.) Inhale and release the contraction.

Repeat at least 20 times each day. Kegels are the most important exercises you will ever do. Many pregnant women who avoid strengthening their pelvic floor muscles experience bowel and bladder problems later in life.

ACKNOWLEDGMENTS

We would like to acknowledge and thank the participants in the Baby & Me—Tobacco Free™ Program who provided questions that needed answering and whose experiences we used when drafting the replies.

Thanks also go to Dr. Anne Gadomski, Dr. John Laird, Dr. Robert Berke, Rocky Mountain Health Foundation, Martha Jones, Lisa Fenton-Free, Michelle Brooks, Barb Hastings, Debra Nichols, Jeff Parnell, Donna Duckworth, Barbara V. Belfie, Lindsay Ball, Kate O'Stricker, John and Cathy Zawacki, George Adams, Nichole Adams, Jared and Ashley Adams Cornell Cooperative Extension of Allegany and Cattaraugus Counties, Gerilee McBride, Bookmasters Inc. Ohio, Brian Feinblum, Tony Proe, Brittany T. Jakubke, M.A. Jakubke, Barbara V. Belfie, and Lesley Cameron. Photograph (Laurie Adams) by Jaime Snyder.

REFERENCES

ABOUT THIS BOOK

1. Baby&Me-Tobacco Free Maternal Child Health Journal 2011 Feb;15(2): 188-97.doi:10-1007/s10995-010-05689. *Effectiveness of a Combined Prenatal and Postpartum Smoking Cessation Program.* Dadomski A, Adams L, Tallman N, Krupa N, Kenkins P. Source Bassett Healthcare Research Institute.

2. Baby&Me http://link.springer.com/article/10.1007%2Fs10995-010-0568-9

3. Baby&Me http://minotdailynews.com/page/content.detail/id/558947/*Drop-it-for-diapers-Pregnant-moms-given-incentive-to-quit-smoking* Pregnant-.html

INTRODUCTION

1. reasons http://www.cdc.gov/reproductivehealth/TobaccoUsePregnancy/

2. reasons http://www.who.int/mediacentre/news/releases/2013/who_ban_tobacco/en/index.html

3. reasons *Maternal smoking during pregnancy and daughter's risk of gestational diabetes and obesity.* K. Mattsson & K. Kallen & M.P. Longnecker & A. Rignell-Hydbom & L. Rylander Diabetologia, May 2013, DOI 10.1007/s00125-013-2936-7

4. reasons *Tobacco Use and Pregnancy*—Centers for Disease Control and Prevention http://www.cdc.gov/reproductivehealth/ tobaccousepregnancy

5. reasons Phillip Quetin *Carcinogens Found in Babies Urine If Their Parents Smoke*, Medical News Today. MediLexicon, Intl, 15 May 2006.

6. doctor Schroeder SA. *How clinicians can help smokers to quit.* JAMA 2012;308:1586-7.

7. doctor http://www.pregnets.org/mothers/*HowToTalk*.aspx

8. anxiety McDermott, M.S. et al. *'Change in anxiety following successful and unsuccessful attempts at smoking cessation: cohort study'* British Journal of Psychiatry. doi:10.1192/bjp.bp.112.114389

9. 95% http://www.quitsolutions.org/New2012HVCCDental.pdf

10. 95% http://lung.ca/_resources/Making_quit_happen_report.pdf and http://whyquit.com/pr/123106/html

11. 30% *Expecting to quit: A best practices review of smoking cessation interventions for pregnant and postpartum women (2nd ed.).* Vancouver: British Columbia Centre of Excellence for Women's Health. Greaves, L., Poole, N., Okoli., C.T.C., Hemsing, N., Qu., A., Bialystok, L., & O'Leary, R. (2011). (Anderka et al., 2010, Crawford, et al., Difranza, et al., 2004; Salmasi, et al., 2010, Klesges, et al., Tong, et al., 2009).

12. **Maternal and Child Health Journal** Maternal Child Health Journal 2011 Feb;15(2): 188-97.doi:10-1007/s10995-010-05689. *Effectiveness of a Combined Prenatal and Postpartum Smoking Cessation Program.* Dadomski A, Adams L, Tallman N, Krupa N, Kenkins P. Source Bassett Healthcare Research Institute.

PART ONE

1. **The Hero Within** by Carol Pearson, Harper One - New York 1998

2. **kid** http://www.tobaccofreekids.org/research/factsheets/pdf/0127.pdf

3. **2013** *21st-Century Hazards of Smoking and Benefits of Cessation in the United States* Prabhat Jha, M.D., Chinthanie Ramasundarahettige, M.Sc., Victoria Landsman, Ph.D., Brian Rostron, Ph.D., Michael Thun, M.D., Robert N. Anderson, Ph.D., Tim McAfee, M.D., and Richard Peto, F.R.S.N Engl J Med 2013; 368:341-350 January 24, 2013DOI: 10.1056/NEJMsa1211128

4. **2013** *50-Year Trends in Smoking-Related Mortality in the United States* Michael J. Thun, M.D., Brian D. Carter, M.P.H., Diane Feskanich, Sc.D., Neal D. Freedman, Ph.D., M.P.H., Ross Prentice, Ph.D., Alan D. Lopez, Ph.D., Patricia Hartge, Sc.D., and Susan M. Gapstur, Ph.D., M.P.H.N Engl J Med 2013; 368:351-364 January 24, 2013 DOI:10.1056/NEJMsa1211127

5. **15% of women** New Evidence That Cigarette Smoking Remains the Most Important Health Hazard, Steven A. Schroeder, M.D. http://smokingcessationleadership.ucsf.edu/sas_nejm_editorial_2013.pdf

6. **Current cigarette smoking among adults**—United States, 2011. MMWR Morb Mortal Wkly Rep 2012;61:889-94.

7. **movies** http://www.surgeongeneral.gov/library/reports/preventing-youth-tobacco-use/exec-summary.pdf

8. **Rihanna** http://www.dailymail.co.uk/tvshowbiz/article-2273534/ *Rihanna-smoulders-plunging-vest-bra-puffs-cigarette-outtakes-photo-shoot.html*

9. **Leonardo DiCaprio** http://smokefreemovies.ucsf.edu/ourads/ad_sfm93.htm

10. **smoking on screen** http://www.smokefreemovies.ucsf.edu/godeeper/the_science.html

11. **Skyfall** http://news.health.com/2012/10/worst-movie-for-smoking December 10, 2012

12. **movies** http://pediatrics.aappublications.org/content/124/1/135. abstract

13. **million an hour** http://www.cnn.com/2012/03/15/health/feds-tobacco-ads

14. **The Cigarette Century The Rise, Fall, and Deadly Persistence of the Product that Defined America** by Allan M. Brandt, Basic Books—New York 2007

15. **children experiment** http://www.dummies.com/how-to/content/preventing-your-teen-from-picking-up-the-smoking-h.html

16. **advertising** World Health Organization 2013 http.who.int/media-centre/news/release/2013/who_ban_tobacco/en/index.html

17. **jumped 34%** http://www.asyousow.org/health_safety/smoking.shtml Lum KL, Polansky JR, Jackler RK, Glantz SA. Signed, sealed, and delivered: Big tobacco in Hollywood, 1927-1951. Tobacco Control 2008 Oct;17(5):313-23

18. **NAAG** http://www.naag.org/movie-studios-should-stop-depicting-smoking-in-youth-rated-movies May 10, 2012

19. **March 8 2012** http://www.cdc.gov/tobacco/data_statistics/sgr/2012/

20. **Teens** http://geiselmed.dartmouth.edu/news/2008/01/14_titus-ernstoff.shtml

21. **movies** http://www.smokefreemovies.ucsf.edu/actnow/

PART TWO Q–I
1. **ashamed** http://www.dailymail.co.uk/femail/article-2001086/Yes-wrong-I-smoked-BOTH-pregnancies-A-regretful-middle-class-mums-confession.html

2. **blame** *Expecting to quit: A best practices review of smoking cessation interventions for pregnant and postpartum women* (2nd ed.). Vancouver: British Columbia Centre of Excellence for Women's Health. Greaves, L., Poole, N., Okoli., C.T.C., Hemsing, N., Qu., A., Bialystok, L., & O'Leary, R. (2011).Page 46

3. **21st. century** *21st-Century Hazards of Smoking and Benefits of Cessation in the United States*—Prabhat Jha, M.D., Chinthanie Ramasundarahettige, M.Sc., Victoria Landsman, Ph.D., Brian Rostron, Ph.D., Michael Thun, M.D., Robert N. Anderson, Ph.D., Tim McAfee, M.D., and Richard Peto, F.R.S.N Engl J Med 2013; 368:341-350January 24, 2013DOI: 10.1056/NEJMsa1211128

4. **21st. century** *50-Year Trends in Smoking-Related Mortality in the United States* Michael J. Thun, M.D., Brian D. Carter, M.P.H., Diane Feskanich, Sc.D., Neal D. Freedman, Ph.D., M.P.H., Ross Prentice, Ph.D., Alan D. Lopez, Ph.D., Patricia Hartge, Sc.D., and Susan M. Gapstur, Ph.D., M.P.H. N Engl J Med 2013; 368:351-364January 24, 2013DOI: 10.1056/NEJMsa1211127

5. **global** http://www.takepart.com/article/2012/08/17/smoking-rates-around-world-are-astronomical

6. **global** http://www.thelancet.com/journals/lancet/article/PIIS0140-6736%2812%2961085-X/fulltext

7. **tobacco industry** http://www.ncbi.nlm.nih.gov/pubmed/20163736

8. **global markets** http://www.huffingtonpost.com/2012/10/09/mitt-romney-bain-tobacco_n_1949812.html

9. **markets** http://www.who.int/tobacco/media/en/TobaccoExplained.pdf

10. **1 billion people** http://www.cdc.gov/tobacco/data_statistics/fact_sheets/fast_facts/

11. **5 million** http://www.cdc.gov/tobacco/data_statistics/fact_sheets/fast_facts/

12. **1 in 5** *http://www.cdc.gov/mmwr/preview/mmwrhtml/mm6144a2.htm*

13. **96 billion** *http://www.cdc.gov/mmwr/preview/mmwrhtml/mm6144a2.htm*

14. **Global Adult** http://www.cnn.com/2012/08/16/health/world-smoking-study

15. **$1 million** http://www.hhs.gov/news/press/2012pres/03/20120308a.html

16. **advertising** http://www.huffingtonpost.com/2012/08/15/australian-cigarette-logo-ban_n_1778145.html

17. **healthcare** http://www.cdc.gov/tobacco/data_statistics/fact_sheets/fast_facts/

18. **tobacco industry** www.thetruth.com

19. **tobacco industry** Volume 114 >> Issue 17 : Friday, April 1, 1994 Tobacco Firm Charged with Suppressing Nicotine Study By William J. Eaton Los Angeles Times *WASHINGTON* http://tech.mit.edu/V114/N17/tobacco.17w.html

20. **tobacco industry** http://www.who.int/tobacco/media/en/ TobaccoExplained.pdf

21. **Garfield Mahood,** *Tobacco Industry Denormalization: Telling the truth about the tobacco industry's role in the tobacco epidemic at* http://www.nsra-adnf.ca/cms/page1381.cfm.

Q-2
1. **attempt** http://www.plosmedicine.org/article/info:doi/10.1371/journal.pmed.1000216

2. **withdrawal** http://whyquit.com/whyquit/a_symptoms.html

3. **withdrawal** http://quitsmoking.about.com/od/cravingsandurges/tp/nicwithdrawalhub.htm

4. **three minutes** http://quitsmoking.about.com/od/cravingsandurges/a/5minutetips.htm

Q-4
1. **quit plan** *The influence of having a quit date on prediction of smoking cessation outcome* Authors James Balmford, Ron Borland and Sue Burney *http://her.oxfordjournals.org/content/25/4/698.full Health Educ. Res. (2010) 25 (4): 698-706. doi: 10.1093/her/cyq013* First published online: March 1, 2010

Q-6
1. **successful quitters** Chapman S, MacKenzie R (2010) *The Global Research Neglect of Unassisted Smoking Cessation: Causes and Consequences.* PLoS Med 7(2): e1000216. doi:10.1371/journal.pmed.1000216

2. **cold turkey** http://whyquit.com/pr/123106.html

3. **3.4%** Cochrane's Review of Abstracts.

4. **single attempts** U.S. Department of Health and Human Services. (2001). *Women and smoking: A report of the Surgeon General.* Atlanta, GA: US Department of Health and Human Services, Centers for Disease Control and Prevention, National Center for Chronic Disease Prevention and Health Promotion, Office on Smoking and Health.

5. **Out On a Limb** January 5th 2013 Seth Godin (Blog)

Q-7
1. **nrt** http://whyquit.com/whyquit/A_OTC_NRT_Meta_Analysis. html

2. **second attempt** Addiction. 1993 Apr;88(4):533-9.*Recycling with nicotine patches in smoking cessation.*Tønnesen P, Nørregaard J, Säwe U, Simonsen K. Source Department of Pulmonary Medicine P, Bispebjerg Hospital, Copenhagen, Denmark

3. **assist with** http://thechart.blogs.cnn.com/2012/01/09/ *study-nicotine-gums-patches-only-help-with-withdrawal/*

4. **nrt** Oncken,C.A. Kranzler, H.R. (2009). *What do we know about the role of pharmacology for smoking cessation before or during pregnancy?* Nicotine and Tobacco Research, 11 (11), 1265-1273

5. **not recommended** The Quick Reference Guide for Clinicians contains strategies and recommendations from the Public Health Service-sponsored Clinical Practice Guideline Treating Tobacco Use and Dependence: 2008 Update Fiore MC, Jaén CR, Baker TB, et al. Treating Tobacco Use and Dependence: 2008 Update. Quick Reference Guide for Clinicians. Rockville, MD: U.S.Department of Health and Human Services. Public Health Service. April 2009.

6. nrt *Promoting Smoking Cessation* MICHELE M. LARZELERE, PhD, and DAVE E. WILLIAMS, MD, Louisiana State University School of Medicine, New Orleans, Louisiana *Am Fam Physician.* 2012 Mar 15;85(6):591-598

7. Harvard http://www.hsph.harvard.edu/news/press-releases/nicotine-replacement-therapies/

8. nrt http://aafp.org/afp/2012/0315/pg591.html diabetes http://www.medicalnewstoday.com/articles/220361.php

9. diabetes http://www.medicalnewstoday.com/articles/220361.php

10. nrt Tob Control doi:10.1136/tobaccocontrol-2011-050129A *prospective cohort study challenging the effectiveness of population-based medical intervention for smoking.* Hillel R Alpert, Gregory N Connolly, Lois Biener.

11. youth, pregnancy, heart disease http://www.webmd.com/*smoking-cessation/nicotine-replacement-therapy-for-quitting-tobacco*

12. nrt http://www.kflapublichealth.ca/Files/Resources/Nicotine_Replacement_Therapy.pdf

13. nrt http://youcanmakeithappen.ca/wp-content/uploads/2011/08/Appendix-C5-Medical-Directive-Public-Health-Unit.pdf

14. nrt http://www.saskcancer.ca/Pharmacotherapy%20Cheat%20Sheet

15. nrt http://theconversation.com/nicotine-replacement-therapy-isnt-all-its-cracked-up-to-be-12153

16. nrt http://whyquit.com/nrt/wsj_helliker_nicotine_fix_020807.html

17. snuff http://www.webmd.com/baby/news/20110826/
snuff-use-during-pregnancy-harmful-to-newborns
18. nrt *Nicotine Damages First Trimester Embryo* http://whyquit.
com/pr/020608.html

Q-8
1. addiction is the cycle http://www.whyquit.com/

2. addiction http://www.quitsolutions.org/New2012HVCCDental.pdf

3. withdrawal http://www.healthline.com/health-slideshow/
quit-smoking-timeline

Q-9
1. one cigarette http://www2.sunysuffolk.edu/benharm/Articles/
hooked%20from%20the%20first%20cigarette.pdf
http://www.tobaccofreekids.org/research/factsheets/pdf/0127.pdf

2. only days http://www.tobaccofreekids.org/research/factsheets/
pdf/0127.pdf

3. brain http://www.ncbi.nlm.nih.gov/pubmed/17004938

4. brian Cosgrove, K.P., et al. ß2-nicotinic acetylcholine receptor
availability during acute and prolonged abstinence from tobacco
smoking. *Archives of General Psychiatry* 66(6): 666-676, 2009

Q-10
1. nature The restorative benefits of nature: Toward an integrative
framework *Journal of Environmental Psychology, Volume 15, Issue 3,
September 1995, Pages 169-182* Stephen Kaplan

2. minds are wandering *Shambhala Sun*, March 2012 Page 46

Q–11

1. **Many women do quit** Int J Occup Med Environ Health. 2005;18(2):159 65. *Smoking relapse one year after delivery among women who quit smoking during pregnancy.* Polańska K, Hanke W, Sobala W. SourceDepartment of Environmental Epidemiology, Nofer Institute of Occupational Medicine, Lódź, Poland. kinga@imp.lodz.pl

Q–12

1. **90%** Chapman S, MacKenzie R (2010) *The Global Research Neglect of Unassisted Smoking Cessation: Causes and Consequences.* PLoS Med 7(2): e1000216. doi:10.1371/journal.pmed.1000216

2. **fascinating** Marsh A, Matheson J (1983) *Smoking behaviour and attitudes.* London: Office of Population Censuses and Surveys. Social Survey Division

3. **believe** Best Health Magazine. *Mixed Messages* Rosemary Counter December 2012 pages 55-56

4. **Spence** Best Health Magazine December 2012 pg. 21

5. **eggs** http://www.thestar.com/life/2012/08/15/egg_yolks_unhealthy_says_western_universitys_david_spence.html

6. **Dr. Serge Rinaud** The Valley Table June-August 2010 *The French Paradox at 20* by Stephen Kolpan

Q–13

1. **Roitfeld** Letter dated September 23, 2011. Addressed to Mr. Brian L. Roberts Chairman and Chief Executive Officer Comcast Corporation from The Secretary of Health and Human Services Washington D.C. Kathleen Sebelius.

2. **Roitfeld** http://www.vogue.com/vogue-daily/article/the-irreverent-carine-roitfeld/#1

3. **Roitfeld** http://fashionista.com/2013/03/carine-roitfeld-breaks-vow-to-never-use-a-ciagarette-in-latest-cr-fashion-book-editorial/

4. **weight** http://www.heartfoundation.org.au/healthy-eating/mums-united/articles/Pages/dont-diet.aspx

5. **Davidoff** http://www.tobaccopub.net/articles/*new-cigarette-brand-davidoff-id-cigarettes* and http://cigarettestimes.com/cigarettes-articles/philip-morris-shares

6. **Master Settlement Agreement** http://www.cdc.gov/mmwr/preview/mmwrhtml/mm6120a3.htm

7. **Harvard School of Public Health** http://www.newscientist.com/article/dn10981-tobacco-pandemic-fuelled-by-nicotine-hike.html **http://archive.sph.harvard.edu/press-releases/2007-releases/press01182007.html**

8. **Harvard School of Public Health** http://archive.sph.harvard.edu/press-releases/2007-releases/press01182007.html

9. **levels** Lewan T. *Dark Secrets of Tobacco Company Exposed.* Tobacco Control. 1997. V.7 315-319

10. *The Cigarette Century The Rise, Fall, and Deadly Persistence of the Product that Defined America* by Allan M. Brandt, Basic Books—New York 2007

11. **The Australia government** http://www.dailymail.co.uk/news/article-2060019/*Australia-country-introduce-unbranded-cigarette-packets*.html

12. **Imperial** http://www.independent.co.uk/news/uk/home-news/*imperial-tobacco-one-of-the-worlds-biggest-cigarette-firms-loses-display-battle*-8411091.html

13. **plain packaging** http://ash.org/*ireland-a-hero-of-tobacco-control*
May 30 2013

14. **plain packaging** http://ash.org/*world-no-tobacco-day-2013-pro-
tecting-public-health-requires- global-effort*/ and http://www.cigaret-
testime.com/cigarettes-articles/philip-morris-shares

15. **Central Park** USA Today Monday May 25th. 2011 page 7A.

16. **Tipalet** http://www.flickr.com/photos/robotbastard/70713561/

17. **N Engl J Med.** 2001 Aug 16;345(7):504-11.*The Master
Settlement Agreement with the tobacco industry and cigarette adver-
tising in magazines.* King C 3rd, Siegel M. Source Harvard Business
School, Boston, MA, USA.

18. **movies** *Behind the Smoke* @Behind_theSmoke (Stanford) Twitter

19. **films** http://www.qdref.org/education/smokescreeners.html *The
impact of On-Screen Smoking in Films*

20. **tobacco industry** http://archive.tobacco.org/resources/history/
tobacco_history20-1.html

21. **tobacco prevention** http://www.who.int/tobacco/publications/
industry/interference/en/

22. **tobacco control** Institute of Medicine of the National Academies.
(2007). *Ending the tobacco problem: A blueprint for the nation* (R.
J Bonnie, K. Stratton, & R.B. Wallace, Eds.). Washington D.C: The
National Academies Press.

23. **scrutiny** March 2004 Garfield Mahood, *Tobacco Industry
Denormalization: Telling the truth about the tobacco industry's role in
the tobacco epidemic at http://www.nsra-adnf.ca/cms/page1381.cfm.*

24. **advertising** http://tobacco.stanford.edu/tobacco_main/index.php

25. **advertising** ASH Action on Smoking & Health. May 30th. 2013 Letter.

Q-14
1. **stimulant** http://smokingaddictionhelp.net/*nicotine-addiction-is-dangerous-for-your-body*.php

Q-15
1. **marijuana** http://www.babycenter.com/404_is-it-safe-to-smoke-marijuana-during-pregnancy_2490.bc

2. **marijuana** http://www.motherisk.org/prof/updatesDetail.jsp?content_id=724

3. **marijuana** http://www.marchofdimes.com/pregnancy/alcohol_illic-itdrug.html

4. **marijuana** http://www.mothertobaby.org/files/marijuana.pdf

5. **marijuana** http://adai.uw.edu/marijuana/factsheets/reproduc-tion.htm Marijuana and Reproduction/Pregnancy. University of Washington

6. **risk** www.otispregnancy.org *Marijuana and Pregnancy*

7. **marijuana** *Reefer Sanity*, Dr. Kevin A. Sabet, Beaufort Books, New York, 2013

Q-17
1. **Gregg Krech** *A Natural Approach to Mental Health* by Gregg Krech, Todo Institute Middlebury, - Vermont 2000.

Q-18

1. **overly** *Willpower*, by Roy F. Baumeister and John Tierney, The Penquin Press – New York 2011

Q-20

1. **brain** http://www.drugabuse.gov/news-events/nida-notes/2009/10/ *abstinent-smokers-nicotinic-receptors-take-more-than-month-to-normalize*

2. **hours** http://www.healthline.com/health-slideshow/ *quit-smoking-timeline#15*

3. **three minutes** http://quitsmoking.about.com/od/cravingsandurges/ a/5minutetips.htm

Q-22

1. **willpower** *Willpower* by Roy F. Baurmeister and John Tierney, The Penguin Press—New York 2011

Q-23

1. **majority** http://lung.ca/_resources/Making_quit_happen_report. pdf

2. **10 years** Campaign For Tobacco-Free Kids: *The Path To Tobacco Addiction Starts At Very Young Ages.*

Q-25

1. **risks** http://www.bbc.co.uk/news/health-22350264

2. **risks** http://www.tobaccofreekids.org/research/factsheets/pdf/0264.pdf

3. **risks** England LJ, Kim SY, Tomar SL, et al. *Non-cigarette tobacco use among women and adverse pregnancy outcomes.* Acta Obstet Gynecol Scand 2010;89:454–64.

4. **risks** http://www.smokefree.gov/healthConsequences/
SmokingHealthConsequencesDescription.aspx

5. **breast milk** Weiser TM, Lin M, Garikapaty V, Feyerham RW,
Bensyl DM & Zhu BP. (2009). *Association of maternal smoking
status with breastfeeding practices*: Missouri, 2005. Pediatrics, 124:
1603-1610.

6. **breastfeeding** http://www.motherisk.org/women/breastfeeding.jsp
Breastfeeding and Drugs

7. **meningitis** http://ash.org/*meningitis-linked-to-smoking-while-pregnant* December 12th. 2012

8. **obesity** http://aje.oxfordjournals.org/content/156/10/954.full

9. **obesity** http://www.dailymail.co.uk/health/article-2197692/
Mothers-smoke-pregnancy-children-risk-obesity-later-on.html

10. **secondhand smoke** www.raisesmokefreekids.com

11. **secondhand smoke** http://www.cdc.gov/tobacco/basic_information/secondhand_smoke/protect_children/index.htm

12. **secondhand smoke** http://jnci.oxfordjournals.org/content/91/5/459.full

13. **secondhand smoke** http://www.cdc.gov/media/releases/2013/
p0516-smoke-free-rules.html

14. **current research** *21st-Century Hazards of Smoking and Benefits
of Cessation in the United States* Prabhat Jha, M.D., Chinthanie
Ramasundarahettige, M.Sc., Victoria Landsman, Ph.D., Brian
Rostron, Ph.D., Michael Thun, M.D., Robert N. Anderson, Ph.D.,
Tim McAfee, M.D., and Richard Peto, F.R.S.N Engl J Med 2013;

368:341-350 January 24, 2013DOI: 10.1056/NEJMsa1211128

15. **current research** *50-Year Trends in Smoking-Related Mortality in the United States* Michael J. Thun, M.D., Brian D. Carter, M.P.H., Diane Feskanich, Sc.D., Neal D. Freedman, Ph.D., M.P.H., Ross Prentice, Ph.D., Alan D. Lopez, Ph.D., Patricia Hartge, Sc.D., and Susan M. Gapstur, Ph.D., M.P.H.N Engl J Med 2013; 368:351-364 January 24, 2013 DOI:10.1056/NEJMsa1211127

16. **current research** *That Cigarette Smoking Remains the Most Important Health Hazard*, Steven A. Schroeder, M.D. http://smokingcessationleadership.ucsf.edu/sas_nejm_editorial_2013.pdf

17. **Jane E. Brody** http://well.blogs.nytimes.com/2013/02/18/ *women-smokers-catch-up/*

Q–26
1. **depression** Boden, J.M., Fergusson, D. M. and Horwood, L. J. *Cigarette smoking and depression: tests of causal linkages using a longitudinal birth cohort. The British Journal of Psychiatry*, Vol. 196, June 2010, pp. 440-46.

2. **depression** Munafo, M. R. and Araya, R. Editorial: *Cigarette smoking and depression: a question of causation. The British Journal of Psychiatry*, Vol. 196, June 2010, pp. 425-26.

3. **depression** Spring, B. et al. Nicotine effects on affective response in depression-prone smokers. *Psychopharmacology*, Vol. 196, February 2008, pp. 461-71.

4. **depression** Schleicher, H. E. et al. *The role of depression and negative affect regulation expectancies in tobacco smoking among college students. The Journal of American College Health*, Vol. 57, March-April 2009, pp. 507-12.

5. **depression** Perkins, K. A. et al. *Acute negative affect relief from smoking depends on the affect situation and measure but not on nicotine. Biological Psychiatry,* Vol. 67, April 2010, pp. 707-14.

6. **depression** http://psychocentral.com/lib/2011/ can-smoking-cause-depression

7. **risk** http://motherisk.org/women/updates *Risks of untreated depression during pregnancy*

Q–27
1. **drinking** *Drunken Compartment* by Craig MacAndrew, Robert B. Edgerton. Percheron Press–New York 2003

2. **alcohol** http://www.acog.org/~/media/For%20Patients/faq170.pdf? dmc=1&ts=20130504T1753352864.

3. **alcohol** The American College of Obstetricians and Gynecologists. www.acog.org/

4. **alcohol** http://www.mothertobaby.org/files/alcohol.pdf

5. **breastfeeding** http://www.marchofdimes.com/baby/feeding_breast-feedingsafe.html

Q–28
1. **e-cigarettes** http://betobaccofree.hhs.gov/about-tobacco/Electronic-Cigarettes/index.html

2. **e-cigarettes** http://www.cdc.gov/media/releases/2013/p0228_electronic_cigarettes.html

3. **e-cigarettes** http://www.cancer.org/healthy/stayawayfromtobacco/ guidetoquittingsmoking/

4. e-cigarettes Williams M, Villarreal A, Bozhilov K, Lin S, Talbot P (2013) *Metal and Silicate Particles Including Nanoparticles Are Present in Electronic Cigarette Cartomizer Fluid and Aerosol*. PLoS ONE 8(3): e57987. doi:10.1371/journal.pone.0057987

5. e-cigarettes http://legacyforhealth.org/newsroom/press-releases/flavored-tobacco-continues-to-play-a-role-in-tobacco-use-among-young-adults

6. e-cigarettes http://tobaccoanalysis.blogspot/ca/2013/04/american-legacy-foundation. *The Rest of the Story: Tobacco News Analysis and Commentary*

Q–31
1. The Four Agreements by Don Miguel Ruiz, Amber-Allen Publishing San Rafael, California. 1997

Q–32
1. reasons http://www.lung.ca/_resources/Appendix_making_quit_happen_provinces.pdf

2. reasons http://www.health.com/health/condition-article/0,,20210803,00.html

3. reasons http://www.john-uebersax.com/diet/nosmoke.htm

4. erectile dysfunction http://www.dailymail.co.uk/femail/article-2292753/*Quit-smoking-Vanity-better-bed-main-reasons-men-smoking-broody-women-quit-conceive*.html

Q–33
1. third-hand smoke https://www.lung.ca/protect-protegez/tobacco-tabagisme/second-secondaire/thirdhand-tertiaire_e.php

2. **third-hand smoke** http://www.mayoclinic.com/health/
third-hand-smoke/ANO1985

3. **second-hand smoke** CDC. The health consequences of smoking:
a report of the Surgeon General. Atlanta, GA: US Department of
Health and Human Services, CDC; 2004. Available at http://www.
cdc.gov/tobacco/data_statistics/sgr/2004/complete_report/index.htm.
Accessed October 24, 2012.

4. **second-hand smoke** http://www.eurekalert.org/pub_
releases/2013-03/acoc-ss030613.php

5. **second-hand smoke** CDC. *The health consequences of involuntary
exposure to tobacco smoke: a report of the Surgeon General.* Atlanta,
GA: US Department of Health and Human Services, CDC; 2006.
Available at http://www.cdc.gov/tobacco/data_statistics/sgr/2006/
index.htm. Accessed October 25, 2012.

6. **second-hand smoke** United Nations. World fertility data 2008.
New York, NY: United Nations, Department of Economic and Social
Affairs, Population Division; 2009. Available at http://www.un.org/
esa/population/publications/WFD%202008/Main.html. Accessed
April 23, 2012.

Q–37
1. **5 to 10%** Centers for Disease Control and Prevention. (2004).
Cigarette smoking among adults-United States,2002. Morbidity and
Mortality Weekly Report, 53(20):427-31 http://www.cdc.gov/repro-
ductivehealth/PrenatalSMKbk/introduction.htm.

2. **succeed** http:dailymail.co.uk/news/article-2060414/Want to quit
smoking?

3. **2007 Youth Risk Behavior Survey** http://www.cdc.gov/mmwr/pre-
view/mmwrhtml/ss5704a1.htm

4. **funding** http://www.tobaccoinfo.ca/mag10/mag10.pdf

5. **funding** http://www.lung.org/about-us/our-impact/top-stories/ *money-at-root-of-nations-tobacco-problem*.html

6. **funding** http://www.tobaccoinfo.ca/mag10/federal.htm

7. **funding** http://ama-assn.org/admednews/2010/12/13/prsa1213. htm *States spending just 2% of tobacco settlement funds on smoking prevention.*

8. **Master Settlement** http://www.cdc.gov/mmwr/preview/mmwrhtml/ mm6120a3.htm

9. **Campaign for Tobacco-Free Kids** http://www.tobaccofreekids.org/ what_we_do/state_local/tobacco_settlement/

10. **tobacco control** News Release Non-smokers Rights Association April 17, 2012. *Big Tobacco Big Winner as Harper Government decimates federal tobacco control strategy.*

11. **children** https://www.gov.uk/government/news/*all-children-really-want-this-christmas-is-their-parents-to-quit-smoking—2*

12. **preventable cause** Fiore,M.C., Jaen, C.R.,Baker,T.B. Bailey, W.C.,Benowitz, N.L., Curry, S.J. et al. (2008). *Treating tobacco use and dependence*: 2008 update. Rockville, MD: US Department of Health and Human Services, US Public Health Service.

Q–40
1. **dads-to-be miss out** http://facet.ubc.ca/wp-content/files/Right-Times-Right-Reasons.pdf

2. **dads-to-be** http://www.fatherhoodinstitute.org/2007/ fatherhood-institute-research-summary-fathers-and-smoking

3. only 33% Fatherhood Institute Research Summary: Fathers and Smoking 20 March 2007 FATHERS AND SMOKING IN THE PERINATAL PERIOD

4. SIDS http://www.cancer.org/cancer/cancercauses/tobaccocancer/ womenand Smoking can affect your baby's health

5. partner Mullen PD.(2004). *How can more smoking suspension during pregnancy become lifelong abstinence? Lessons learned about predictors, interventions, and gaps in our accumulated knowledge.* Nicotine & Tobacco Research, 6(Suppl2):S217-S238. US Department of Health and Human Services 2010, Solomon LJ Higgins ST, Heil SH, Badger GJ, Thomas CS, Bernstein IM. *Predictors of postpartum relapse to smoking.* Drug and Alcohol Dependence 2007;90(2-3):224-7

6. dads-to-be Bottorff, J.L. Kalaw, C., Johnson, J.L., Chambers, N., Stewart, M., Greaves, L.,& Kelly, M. (2005) Unravelling smoking ties: How tobacco use is embedded in couple interactions. *Research in Nursing and Health*, 28(4), 316-328

7. dads-to-be Oliffe, J.L., Bottorff, J.L., & Sarbit, G. (2012). Mobilizing masculinity to support fathers who want to be smoke free. CIHR Institute of Gender and Health Knowledge Translation Casebook. Ottawa, ON: CIHR.

8. Dr.Margaret Chan http.who.int/mediacentre/news/release/2013/ who_ban_tobacco/en/index.html

9. tobacco statistics and facts http://ash.org/resources/ tobacco-statistics-facts/

INDEX

A Message to Healthcare Providers:
The Clinical Practice Guideline—Health and Human Services (2008 update) CDC—Treating Tobacco Use and Dependence contains strategies and recommendations designed to assist clinicians, tobacco dependence treatment specialists, healthcare administrators, insurers, and providers in delivering and supporting effective treatments for tobacco use and dependence. Tobacco dependence is a chronic disease that often requires repeated intervention and multiple attempts to quit. However, effective treatments exist and can significantly increase rates of long-term abstinence. It is essential that clinicians and healthcare delivery systems consistently identify and document tobacco-use status and treat every tobacco user they see in a healthcare setting.

A Message to the Reader:
This book is for educational purposes and is not intended to replace the advice of your family physician or other healthcare provider. The purchaser or reader of this book hereby acknowledges receiving notice of this DISCLAIMER. The authors and Grafton and Scratch Publishers are not engaged in providing medical care or services, and the information presented in this book is in no way intended to be treated as medical advice or as a substitute for medical counseling. The information in this book is not intended to diagnose or treat any medical or physical condition or problem. This book is based upon information taken from sources believed to be reliable. The reader should use this book only as a general guide. Those who read this book acknowledge that they are relying upon their own investigation and not on any statements or opinions expressed herein and are